Person-Centre

Patient Centred Nursing

Person-Centred Nursing
Theory and Practice

Brendan McCormack
Professor of Nursing Research
Institute of Nursing Research/School of Nursing
University of Ulster
Northern Ireland

Tanya McCance
Mona Grey Professor for Nursing R&D
Institute of Nursing Research/School of Nursing
University of Ulster & Co-Director – Nursing R&D
Belfast Health & Social Care Trust
Northern Ireland

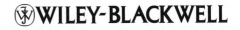

A John Wiley & Sons, Ltd., Publication

This edition first published 2010
© Brendan McCormack and Tanya McCance

Blackwell Publishing was acquired by John Wiley & Sons in February 2007. Blackwell's publishing programme has been merged with Wiley's global Scientific, Technical, and Medical business to form Wiley-Blackwell.

Registered office
John Wiley & Sons Ltd, The Atrium, Southern Gate, Chichester, West Sussex, PO19 8SQ, United Kingdom

Editorial office
9600 Garsington Road, Oxford, OX4 2DQ, United Kingdom
2121 State Avenue, Ames, Iowa 50014-8300, USA

For details of our global editorial offices, for customer services and for information about how to apply for permission to reuse the copyright material in this book please see our website at www.wiley.com/wiley-blackwell.

Library of Congress Cataloging-in-Publication Data
McCormack, Brendan.
  Person-centred nursing : theory and practice/Brendan McCormack, Tanya McCance.
     p.; cm.
  Includes bibliographical references and index.
  ISBN 978-1-4051-7113-7 (pbk.: alk. paper)
  1. Nurse and patient. 2. Nursing—Psychological aspects. I. McCance, Tanya. II. Title.
  [DNLM: 1. Holistic Nursing—methods. 2. Nurse-Patient Relations. 3. Outcome Assessment (Health Care) 4. Patient Participation. 5. Patient Satisfaction. WY 86.5 M4778p 2010]
  RT86.3.M43 2010
  610.7306′99—dc22
                                                                                                    2010007730

A catalogue record for this book is available from the British Library.

Set in 9.5/11.5pt Sabon by MPS Limited, A Macmillan Company, Chennai, India
Printed and bound in Great Britain by TJ International Ltd, Padstow, Cornwall

3   2012

Contents

Author Biographies

Brendan McCormack, DPhil (Oxon.), BSc (Hons.) Nursing, PGCEA, RNT, RMN, RGN

Professor of Nursing Research, Institute of Nursing Research/ School of Nursing, University of Ulster, Northern Ireland; Adjunct Professor of Nursing, University of Technology, Sydney; Adjunct Professor of Nursing, Faculty of Medicine, Nursing and Health Care, Monash University, Melbourne.

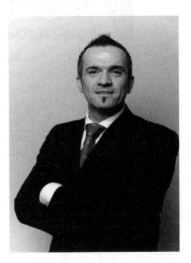

Brendan is professor of Nursing Research and Director of the Institute of Nursing Research, University of Ulster. He leads and contributes to a number of practice development and research projects in Ireland, the UK, Europe, Canada and Australia that focus on the development of person-centred practice. In addition, he is the Head of the 'Person-Centred Practice Research Centre' in the Institute of Nursing Research, coordinating research and development activity in this area. His writing and research work focuses on gerontological nursing, person-centred nursing and practice development, and he serves on a number of editorial boards, policy committees and development groups in these areas. His most recent work has been leading the development of the 'Northern Ireland Single Assessment Tool' for older people in Northern Ireland – unique to the UK, because of its integrated health and social care foundation. He has a particular focus on the use of arts and creativity in healthcare research and development. Brendan has more than 100 peer-reviewed publications as well as 6 books published and in progress. He is the editor of the 'International Journal of Older People Nursing'. He has co-authored *Practice Development in Nursing* which has now been translated into two languages and *Practice Development in Nursing: International Perspectives (published 2008)*. Brendan is President of the All-Ireland Gerontological Nurses Association [AIGNA] and Chairman of the charity 'Age NI'.

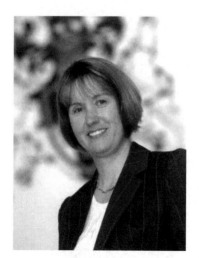

Tanya McCance, DPhil, MSc, BSc (Hons.), RGN
Mona Grey Professor for Nursing Research and Development, Institute of Nursing Research/School of Nursing, University of Ulster and Co-Director – Nursing R&D, Belfast Health and Social Care Trust, Northern Ireland.

Tanya is professor for Nursing R&D, which is a joint appointment between the University of Ulster and the Belfast Health and Social Care Trust. She has been a registered nurse since 1990 and throughout her career has held several joint posts demonstrating her commitment to practice, education and research. Tanya currently leads a number of projects that are practice based and collaborative in nature, which contribute to a programme of work that focuses on person-centred care. Her interest is in developing research in practice and a lot of her work would be in this context. Tanya currently sits on a number of editorial boards, committees and working groups and is recognised for her contribution to the strategic development of nursing and midwifery R&D. Her CV reflects her interests, with over 20 publications (full papers and book chapters) and delivery of a range of regional, national and international conference presentations. Her most recent work focuses on the identification of a relevant and appropriate set of key performance indicators for nursing and midwifery that are indicative of person-centred care and the development of methodologies that will demonstrate the contribution of nursing to the patient experience.

Acknowledgements

Ambitions new and vibrant
Energising plans
Sustaining joint venturing

The 'Haiku' above reflects the essence of the experience of writing this book. Like all authors we set off with ambitious plans for how we would write, achieve our deadlines and targets and create an exciting text that we have talked about for a long time. We have been colleagues and friends for ten years and together have shaped and reshaped each others' thinking about person-centredness and how it manifests itself in practice, education, research and practice development. Like all 'duos' we have our complementary strengths, and our work reflects the trust in each others commitment and dedication to a vision for developing person-centred practice, which has carried us through the journey that has resulted in this book.

We have not been alone in this experience and there are many people who have helped and encouraged us along the way – to these people we are eternally grateful, you know who you are and we thank you sincerely for your support, friendship, colleagueship, challenge and generosity. In particular we would like to thank Neil, Mark and Melissa (and their grandparents), Lorna, Michael, Aideen and Fionn for the love, support, encouragement and care you have shown to us in making this project happen and seeing it to fruition. We are grateful for the conditions you provided in enabling our writing and hopeful that you will forgive us for the lost hours away from you!

Many people have contributed examples from their work, have provided us with stories and tales of personal experiences, have volunteered to write case examples for us to use and have provided critical commentary as the chapters evolved. We would like to thank, programme participants in the Republic of Ireland Older Persons National Practice Development Programme, programme participations from the Belfast Trust's PCC Programme, Dr Jan Dewing, Dr Angie Titchen, Michele Hardimann, Shaun Cardiff, Marie-Louise van Hest, Lorna Peelo-Kilroe, Heidi Dowse, Philip Eldridge,

Julie Farmer, Tamra MacLeod, Carmel Gibbons, Anna-Marie Harmon, Bernadette Gribben, Christine Boomer, Dr Paul Slater, Valerie Jackson, Moira Davren, Randal Parlour and Ann Coyne-Nevin.

Finally, we would like to thank our colleagues at Wiley-Blackwell for encouraging us along the way and forgiving the missed deadlines. Your confidence in the final product has helped us stay the course.

Brendan McCormack and Tanya McCance

Chapter 1

Introduction

Person-centred care has a long association with nursing, and at a level of principle is well understood as that which is concerned with: treating people as individuals; respecting their rights as a person; building mutual trust and understanding, and developing therapeutic relationships. As nurses we have an expectation that people should receive a standard of care that reflects these principles. The inherent good of providing care within a philosophy of person-centredness is irrefutable, but it has been recognised that translating the core concepts into every day practice is challenging (McCormack & McCance, 2006). The reasons for this come in many forms and are often indicative of the context in which care is being delivered, and the fact that we are living in times of constant change, particularly within health and social care.

The promotion of 'person-centredness' is consistent with international policy developments and is reflected in approaches to the delivery of healthcare. Within the United Kingdom, person-centredness is embedded in many policy initiatives such as *The National Service Framework for Older People* (DoH, 2001a) and the *Dignity in Care Campaign* (DoH, 2006). Furthermore, from a professional perspective, there is a desire to reaffirm the importance of the fundamentals of care, emphasised by the recent publication of a report by the Royal College of Nursing (RCN) (2008), which highlights the challenges for nurses and midwives in providing sensitive and dignified care. Similarly, within a Northern Ireland context there has been an increasing emphasis on improving the service user experience (DHSSPS, 2008), where the focus is explicitly on the promotion of person-centred standards across the health and social care sector. The drive, however, within the health service to demonstrate effectiveness and efficiency through performance management processes has never been greater. This has resulted in a range of quality and clinical indicators, which pay little attention to how patients, clients and their families experience care (DHSSPS, 2007a; Nolan, 2007). Whilst nurses have a significant contribution to make in determining the quality of care provided to patients/clients and their families, a review of the evidence reveals a greater emphasis on areas of nursing and midwifery practice that can be quantified, for example, pressure ulcer incidence, rates of healthcare associated infection and incidence of falls generally referred to as metrics. In contrast, there are fewer indicators that are person-centred in their orientation, which can evidence the impact of nursing and midwifery care on the patient experience (National Nursing Research Unit, 2008). In this context, we would argue that the time is ripe for promoting new ways of working that can deliver effective person-centred practice, and using approaches that can demonstrate positive outcomes as a result.

Whilst the term 'person-centred' care is most often seen in the UK health and social care literature and policy documents, the foci that underpin person-centred care are synonymous with international movements that focus on humanising the health and social care experience. For example, in 1994 Wagner reported on action research that focused on integrated health and social care for older people in relation to preventative work and ensuring that residents in care homes had the same rights as citizens in society (Wagner, 1994). The 'Skaevinge Project' model as it became known influenced the future shape of residential care and the design of care homes internationally. Principles such as autonomy, citizenship, dignity and respect (that also underpin principles of person-centred care) are central to this model and ways of working. Healthcare policy around the world embraces these same principles and underpins many policy frameworks for health and social care. For example, in Australia the 'Aged Care Standards and Accreditation Agency' have principles of person-centred care as a central building block of facility accreditation. Whilst the New South Wales Nursing Department has a focus on developing practices and models of care to support person-centredness across all specialities. This is important to emphasise, as for many professionals, person-centred care is often seen as being synonymous with older-person care/services. Whilst the majority of literature has focused on older people, mainly because of the influences of early writers/researchers such as Tom Kitwood, person-centred care is not exclusive to older people. Developing models of care that enable person-centred principles to be realised across all services is a key issue in health and social care reform. Most notably is the influence of the 'Institute for Healthcare Improvement (IHI)' in the United States of America. The transformation of health and social care services is a focus of many western governments and many of the innovation frameworks and tools have emanated from the IHI. The focus of much of the work is on the development of person-centred care mainly through the transformation of healthcare systems, structures and the redesign of clinical services.

Also, there is a growing empirical evidence base that focuses on person-centredness as highlighted from a comprehensive literature review undertaken by McCormack (2004). This review identified a total of 110 papers that related to aspects of person-centred practice research. In summary, research into person-centredness has attempted to clarify the meaning of the term (e.g. McCormack, 2004), explore the implications of the term in practice (Dewing, 2004) and determine the cultural and contextual challenges to implementing a person-centred approach (Binnie & Titchen, 1999; McCormack et al., 2008b). Whilst a number of conceptual frameworks for person-centred nursing exist (e.g. Binnie & Titchen, 1999; McCormack, 2001b, 2003, 2004; Nolan et al., 2004), there are few studies that enhance our understanding of how we can effectively operationalise person-centredness in practice, or evaluate the relationship between a person-centred approach to nursing and the resulting outcomes for patients and nurses. The Person-Centred Nursing Framework (McCormack & McCance, 2006) described in this book has been developed as a tool to facilitate nurses to explore person-centred care in their practice. We believe the Framework can provide a lens that enables the operationalisation of person-centred care and can be used to evaluate developments in practice and hence demonstrate outcomes.

The Person-Centred Nursing Framework

The Person-Centred Nursing (PCN) Framework was developed by McCormack and McCance (2006) and was derived from previous empirical research focusing on person-centred practice with older people (McCormack, 2001) and the experience of caring in nursing (McCance et al., 2001). In summary, the original framework comprised the following four constructs:

1. *Prerequisites*, which focus on the attributes of nurse and include: being professionally competent; having developed interpersonal skills; being committed to the job; being able to demonstrate clarity of beliefs and values; and knowing self.
2. *Care environment*, which focuses on the context in which care is delivered and includes: appropriate skill mix; systems that facilitate shared decision-making; effective staff relationships; organisational systems that are supportive; the sharing of power; and the potential for innovation and risk taking.
3. *Person-centred processes*, which focus on delivering care through a range of activities and include: working with patient's beliefs and values; engagement; having sympathetic presence; sharing decision-making; and providing for physical needs.
4. *Outcomes*, the central component of the Framework, are the results of effective PCN and include: satisfaction with care; involvement in care; feeling of well-being; and creating a therapeutic environment.

The relationship between the constructs suggest that in order to deliver positive outcomes for both patients and staff, account must first be taken of the prerequisites, which impact on the nurses' ability to manage the care environment and the care environment, which in turn are necessary for providing effective care through person-centred processes.

This book aims to provide a more comprehensive explanation of the four constructs that comprise the Person-Centred Nursing Framework and the core elements within each construct. It is useful, however, at the outset to highlight some issues that will enhance understanding for the reader.

- The following terminology used within the Framework requires clarification to ensure accurate interpretation:
  - *person* refers to all those involved in a caring interaction and therefore encompasses patients, clients, families/carers, nursing colleagues and other members of the multidisciplinary team
  - *patient* is the term used throughout for ease of reading, but denotes *patients, clients, families, carers*
- Since our original publication we have continued to test the Framework in practice with a view to further refinement. As a result of this activity we have made the following two changes:
  - added the physical environment as an additional element to the care environment construct in recognition of the impact of our physical surroundings on person-centred practice
  - amended 'providing for physical needs' to read 'providing holistic care', in recognition of the range of interventions undertaken by nurses that are not always physical in nature.

  (The amended Framework is presented in Chapter 3.)
- The four constructs and elements within the Framework, whilst presented separately, are interconnected. One idea is often closely related to another and there will be many examples of this highlighted throughout the book. As a consequence we will often cross reference enabling the reader to make important connections.

Structure of the Book

This book is presented in seven sequential chapters, with each chapter building on previous chapters. Chapters 2 and 3 are philosophical, theoretical and conceptual in their content, and whilst potentially complex, are important in terms of understanding the origins of the Framework and its development. Chapters 4–7 focus on each of the four constructs and attempt to promote an understanding of elements within each construct in context of the existing evidence and through practice examples. The final chapter draws on real projects from practice that have used the Person-Centred Nursing Framework in a variety of different ways, but with the common aim of promoting person-centred cultures.

We have written this book with a broad target audience in mind, and have tried to ensure that it is accessible to nurses working at different levels. We believe the use of stories should help accomplish this goal. It is important to acknowledge that some stories presented are drawn from the published literature, whilst others are 'factions' (fiction that draws on personal experience). We have also tried to ensure the patient's voice is heard throughout, hence the use of extracts, which again have been drawn from a variety of sources. Finally, in the sprit of critical reflection we have peppered throughout the book some 'thoughts to ponder', which are presented as reflective questions. We hope this activity will provide personal insights that lead to new and exciting discoveries about PCN.

Chapter 2
Personhood and Person-Centredness

Introduction

In this chapter we aim to explore the concepts of personhood and person-centredness as they relate to the theory and practice of PCN. As we have reiterated from the outset, whilst PCN may be an increasingly familiar term, the reality is that it is a complex term with many and varied meanings and understandings. Part of the complexity of the term is its philosophical underpinnings, that is the concept of being a 'person'. In philosophy, there are as many differing perspectives on the meaning of 'person' as there are their applications in practice. These differing philosophical perspectives have shaped the way in which the theoretical frameworks have developed and the way these frameworks are applied in practice. This chapter will explore the concepts of 'person' and personhood. It will then develop the idea of 'being an authentic person' as a unifying concept in person-centredness.

The Concept of 'Person'

In everyday life, for most people the word 'person' is used merely as the singular version of 'people'. However, the word 'person' is of greater interest than this, and instead it aims to capture those attributes that represent our humanness and the way in which we construct our way of life. How we think about moral values, how we express political, spiritual or religious beliefs and how we engage emotionally and in relationships are all shaped by our attributes as persons. However, what these attributes are and how they relate to each other is widely debated. Whatever way we explore the issue of 'person' there are no black-and-white positions. However, in this chapter we are concerned with how the concept of person relates to that of 'personhood' and thus our exploration is limited by this intent. We suggest four different perspectives, each of which offers a different lens on the concept of person and ultimately each shapes the way person-centredness is operationalised in practice – an attributes perspective, a reflective perspective, a moral perspective and an embodied perspective. These are not mutually exclusive perspectives and our concluding section will draw upon all these in order to highlight the importance of 'authenticity' as a core concept in person-centredness.

A Hierarchy of Attributes

The word 'person' has been debated for as long as philosophical thought has existed. How we distinguish between persons and other species (such as animals) is a key debate within this long tradition and one that underpins many moral and ethical frameworks. For example, animal-rights advocates and campaigners would argue vehemently that it is morally wrong for pharmaceuticals and cosmetics to be tested on animals before they are used with humans. Their argument would be predicated on the belief that humans and animals are equal and thus should be treated equally. For others, humans are considered to be a higher order species to animals, and thus it is reasonable to use animals in this way in order to benefit the greater good of persons. The position taken in such debates would in part be influenced by views about what it means to be a person. However, even within the 'human species' a person may mean different things, so for example, debates about abortion are influenced by different ideas about whether or not an embryo is a person; is a foetus a person or when does a foetus becomes a person? And indeed if a human being with certain kinds of brain damage/disorders (such as severe head injury or dementia) can be bestowed with the status of 'person'?

For some philosophers (Frankfurt, 1989) it is not enough to claim that human beings are persons on the basis of a collection of physical and psychological attributes because it is conceptually possible that members of another species could lay claim to personhood. If attributes such as sight, taste, smell, sexuality, memory, desires, motives, etc., were to be used as a means of classifying persons from non-persons, then we could easily provide a list of members of other species who would possess similar attributes. Further, the loss of some of these attributes (e.g. a person with dementia may experience deterioration of memory and motivation) would mean that a person could legitimately lose the status of person. Indeed even such higher order attributes as 'thought' and decision-making fail to distinguish persons from other creatures. Human beings are not alone in having desires and preferences. Members of other species share these attributes with human beings and some species could even be seen to base action on deliberation and even prior thought. Think about how a lion living in the wild, plans the killing of his prey – much deliberation, 'thought' and sophisticated decision-making goes into the setting up of the conditions to enable a successful kill to occur. Similarly, if we believe that the possession of a language distinguishes us as persons, then of course studies of animal communication patterns would suggest that different animal species have their own unique language. Further, the loss of language (e.g. arising from certain brain injury) could also mean the loss of the status of person.

It can be seen therefore that distinguishing persons from non-persons on the basis of a hierarchy of attributes is problematic. Some authors, such as Post (2006), argue that a dominant focus in Western cultures on some attributes being more important than others has led to a position whereby cognitive attributes of persons are given greatest importance. Thus, the loss of these attributes can have significant impact on human beings and their personhood (e.g. people with dementia).

The Reflective Person

From this perspective, our uniqueness as humans is distinguished by our ability to engage in reflection on our actions. It is the ability to engage in reflective evaluation of action that distinguishes persons from non-persons. Other creatures are able to have the capacity for what Frankfurt (1989) refers to as 'first-order desires', that is 'desires to do or not to do one thing or another'. But according to Frankfurt, it is a peculiar human trait to not just *want*, choose or be moved to action, but to also *want* to have (or not to have) certain desires and motives. Persons are capable of wanting to be different in their preferences and purposes from what they are, that is 'second-order desires' or 'desires of the second order' (Frankfurt, 1989). Through this reflection, an individual is able to derive a set of principles to guide choices about what should be done in particular situations.

> Robert, aged 25, lives with his partner and 3-year-old son. Robert is increasingly aware of his anger and sometimes inability to control his anger. He has not been physically aggressive towards his partner or his son, but he is scared that sometimes he has the desire to be physically aggressive and is afraid of this happening. Robert knows that his father had a tendency to 'lash out' and he experienced his beatings and violent rows between his father and mother. Robert is very anxious that he doesn't repeat these patterns. He seeks help to understand the basis of his anger and learns strategies for managing it. These strategies are based on principles of emotional management and understanding these principles helps Robert to avoid aggressive outbursts and feel better about himself as a person.

Having a 'want' is a complex issue and sometimes in discussions of autonomy, 'wanting to do' this or that is often seen as the hallmark of being an autonomous person. Being free and acting autonomously is often seen as being able to do what one wants to do. What this description misses is the notion of the *will*. Animals (who are free) can run in whatever direction they wish. Therefore having the freedom to act is a sufficient condition of being free, but not a necessary one. The freedom to make a free choice would be seen as 'negative freedom' by Berlin (1992). Berlin outlines two differing concepts of 'freedom' – *negative freedom:* being free to do what one wants to do *or* 'freedom from' (suppression, *for example*) and *positive freedom:* the freedom to live a prescribed form of life *or* 'freedom to' make decisions as a thinking, willing, active being, bearing responsibility for one's own choices and being able to explain them through reference to one's own ideas and purposes.

> I wish to be an instrument of my own, not other men's acts of will. I wish to be a subject, not an object. . . . deciding, not being decided for, self-directed and not acted upon by external nature or by other men as if I were a thing, or an animal, or a slave incapable of playing a human role, that is, of conceiving goals and policies of my own and realising them.
>
> (Berlin, 1992: 131)

Berlin's idea of a person is one of being self-determined, contributing to and co-creating the social world and doing this through the making of rational choices and reflection on second-order desires. Even though a person may be no longer free to do what he [*sic*] wants to do (because of a disabling illness *for example*) his *'will'* may remain as free as he was before. Although the person cannot turn his desires into actions, he is still free to form those desires and determine possible actions as freely as if his freedom of action had not been impaired (Frankfurt, 1989: 70).

This is particularly important when we consider people who have a dementia or cognitive impairment. Whilst a person with severe dementia may not be able to act independently, the person still has desires that can be enacted with assistance and thus it is important to try to understand these desires (Dewing, 2008a).

Margaret lives with her partner in a Scottish City. Margaret has advanced stage multiple sclerosis with motor and coordination symptoms. Recently, she has started to experience deterioration in her memory and is becoming increasingly dysphasic. Margaret has always had a very active social life and she had a well-established social routine that resulted in her meeting people and attending clubs most days of the week. She was vice president of the widows and widowers club in her local area until recently when she has had to give up this role. She expresses a lot of frustration about that. Margaret's family is concerned about her increasing social isolation as she knows few of her neighbours anymore and her inability to engage in conversation adds to this isolation. Margaret's partner lacks confidence in supporting her to retain her previous level of social engagement and is fearful of placing Margaret in situations that may cause her harm. Margaret, however, has little desire to give up her social connections and expresses the desire to carry on with many of these. She does this by continuing to adhere to her previous routines and at certain times of the day will get ready to attend a club as she has always done. However, she cannot do so independently. A multidisciplinary assessment of her needs, a carer's assessment and discussion with her family are undertaken and a plan of health and social care support/assistance is put in place for Margaret and her partner that enables her to continue to have a full and active social life.

Having a free will is not about the relationship between what one does and what one wants to do, but rather it is about the right to be treated as a person, as the owner of one's own body, as the owner of one's own decisions and as the maker of choices.

The Intrinsic Moral Good of Persons

Immanuel Kant appeared to be quite clear about the notion of 'person' when he stated, 'Act in such a way that you always treat humanity, whether in your own person or in the person of any other, never simply as a means, but always at the same time as an end' (Paton, 1964).

In differentiating between persons and things, Kant suggests that if things have any value at all, then it is merely extrinsic value. That is, things (whether of natural or artificial origin) are only regarded as artificially good, insofar as someone happens to desire them and regard them as valuable. It follows that things have a price, that is their value is determined by the price that someone is willing to pay for them; and as artifacts can be exchanged for things of equal or relative value then it clearly has no unique, absolute, intrinsic worth. If things can be measured in terms of money, then money is regarded as the ultimate standard of value (Sullivan, 1990). What though, does it mean for persons to exist 'as an end in themselves'? As Kant explains, things and animals are only contingently desired (or feared) by and so possibly valued (or given a negative value) by someone. Kant argues that whilst persons have conditional value, such as being nice, good, likeable, loveable or useful, persons should always be regarded as having objective, absolute and intrinsic worth, whether or not they also happen to be valued because they contribute to another's happiness. But one can imagine situations where people are not treated as their own end – treatment decisions based on cost rather than on effects on individual quality of life, the attribution of salary to particular work roles and social class division, are examples of people not being treated as their own end. For example, the potential for older people and people with learning disabilities to be treated as a 'thing' is great, given the potential impact of institutionalisation (Goffman, 1961). McCormack (2001b) highlighted this potential in a composite reflection of his early practice experience.

It's 1980. John has Alzheimer's disease and post-war trauma. He sits in his emaciated frail body in a large, open dormitory, tied to his 'Buxton Chair' with a bed sheet, eating porridge, most of which he spills down his chest – a chest that is exposed because there aren't any buttons in his shirt – a shirt that I had earlier put on him from the communal clothes cupboard. John continues to spill his porridge as it piles up on his lap and little of it gets past his lips because of the tardive dyskinesia[1] he has developed from over prescribing of chlorpromazine to 'keep him quiet'. "You're a demented old bastard" shouts Eamon the staff nurse as he scoops the spilled porridge from John's lap and puts it back in the bowl. John stares. "You're a demented old bastard" shouts Eamon again. John screams. Eamon puts porridge in John's open, screaming mouth until it pours out of his mouth again. John screams a gargled scream as he spits porridge. Eamon hits him. John screams. Eamon wheels him to a side ward and locks the door. John screams . . . from a distance. I keep myself busy by making beds and trying to block out the reality of what is happening. I take John from his faeces and urine soiled conditions, as fortunately it is his bath day. The charge nurse gives him Chlorpromazine in case he 'misbehaves' again as Eamon has reported his version of events. I take John's clothes off and he sits in his emaciated naked body in an open corridor, among 5 other naked men who all wait their turn in the bathroom. I stand with them and make sure they stay in line and don't wander off – I'm powerful in my post, like a soldier on sentry duty, and I need to impress the charge nurse as I'm fed up making beds. A ward domestic walks past John and makes a sound into John's ear that resembles a "bomb exploding". John screams, slouches in his chair and bites his clenched fist. The charge nurse shouts at me for allowing John to scream. The domestic laughs and walks away. John has his bath – I wheeled him in, Eamon poured water on him – John screamed, Eamon laughs, Liam (another staff nurse who prefers playing rugby) whisks John's emaciated body from the bath, dries him roughly and passes him back to me to dress him – a clean shirt and trousers, but funny, this shirt has no buttons either. John and I sit on the ward verandah. It's peaceful here. John sits upright in his chair, no bed sheet as a restraint and he seems to be looking around. The charge nurse shouts – it's time to make the beds again.

(McCormack, 2001: 213)

It is because of being under the moral law that each and every person has an intrinsic, inalienable, unconditional, objective worth or dignity as a person. By virtue of that law we are elevated above being merely part of the natural world. We have an absolute and irreplaceable worth for our value is not dependent on our usefulness or desirability. It has no price or no equivalent for which the object of esteem could be exchanged. We may never renounce our right to respect, and we ought never act in such a way as to reduce either ourselves or others to the status of mere things.

(Sullivan, 1990: 197)

This plea to the intrinsic moral good of persons represents a universal moral principle that extends beyond individual attributes and social, cultural or behavioural characteristics of persons. Everyone desires to lead a good life and therefore has the capacity to reason morally. Freedom of the will does not mean the freedom to do whatever one wants as a free agent. Instead, moral considerations need to be made. Freedom of the will is a moral freedom, based on a world view where the person can '. . . identify with his motivating influences, assimilates them to himself, views himself as a kind of person who wishes to be moved in particular ways and that these influences are the ones he wishes to be identified with' (Dworkin, 1989).

In the chapter so far, it could be concluded that in order to be a person there is a need to engage in rational reflective thought and without this one cannot hold the status of 'person'. Thus, it could be argued that the 'body' is irrelevant to being a person and that it is our mind that matters, that is there is a hierarchical relationship between mind and body. This reinforces a mind–body duality and raises serious challenges to the personhood of people who aren't able (for a host of reasons) to engage in rational reflection about their existence in the world.

The Embodied Person and Personhood

To some extent, Tom Kitwood (1997) was challenging this mind–body hierarchical relationship when he argued that being a person meant to have 'personhood' and that personhood is:

> . . . a standing or status that is bestowed upon one human being, by 'others', in the context of relationship and social being. It implies recognition, respect and trust.
>
> (1997: 8)

However, Kitwood's view still has conditions attached to personhood, that is it is dependent on others recognising one's status as a person and it only exists in relationship with others. Kitwood argues that persons don't exist in isolation, but instead we each have a 'context' in which our personhood is manifested. Kitwood's definition of personhood is informed by the work of Swiss psychologist Paul Tournier (1999) and the philosophies of Martin Buber (1984) and Carl Rogers (1961). Kitwood's work has been highly influential in the world of dementia care and this is understandable as a convincing argument is presented by Kitwood as to why people should be respected for their intrinsic worth even if they can no longer engage in rational reflection on action because of debilitating changes to the brain/mind.

The influence of Kitwood's work can be seen to extend beyond the boundaries of dementia care and Dewing (2008c) argues that the definition of personhood offered by Kitwood has influenced the way in which person-centredness is generally conceptualised in nursing, but that this is often done from a narrow or poor understanding of

Kitwood's work. In a critique of Kitwood's work and a representation of his core ideas, Dewing highlights the importance of 'embodiment' in Kitwood's original ideas, but these were never fully developed in his concept of personhood and person-centred dementia care. Whilst Kitwood has been criticised (Adams, 1996; Nolan et al., 2004) for an individualistic notion of persons and in particular the privileging of the individualised relationship with the person with dementia, Dewing (2008) argues that critics of Kitwood have failed to see the importance of 'others' in his work. Persons don't exist in isolation but exist in relationship with and to others.

Merleau-Ponty (Dillon, 1988) argues that the person 'is the body' and that we exist through bodily engagement with the world. Thus, the body is 'our expression in the world, the visible form of our intentions' (Baldwin, 2004: 36). Mental and physical properties are inseparable, each intertwined with the other creating a seamless whole (Edwards, 2001). Thus our existence is constituted by our 'being in the world', by the relationship between 'our body and the world, between ourselves and our body'. Edwards (2001) argues that thinking about person's from the perspective of 'body' enables us to think about illness and disability in different ways and in the case of (for example) people with dementia or severe physical or mental disabilities, makes a significant contribution to understanding how the personhood of such a person can be retained, by paying attention to bodily responses in the absences of rational reflective abilities.

Jan Dewing's (2007) research into older people with dementia who 'wander' provides us with excellent examples of embodied personhood. Through the video-analysis and dialogues of 10 older people who reside in care homes and who wander, Dewing showed how even when apparent rational thought and reflection was absent, these people were seen to have feelings including desires and to make choices pertaining to their wandering activities and appreciation of wandering.

Dewing thus argues that no understanding of persons can be complete without paying attention to concepts of being, space and time. Specifically with wandering, Dewing (2007) suggests wandering is:

> the embodied manifestation of the ways in which a person living with an advancing dementia actively creates integrated meanings encompassing relationships with 'me', others and objects within named spaces and lived time.

More broadly, and still drawing on Merleau-Ponty's ideas, Dewing argues and demonstrates that there are four fundamental life-world themes (or existentials) that constitute lived experience. These existentials provide helpful 'discovery guides' for reflecting on personhood and lived experiences. The four existentials are: lived body (corporeality), lived human relation (relationality), lived space (spatiality) and lived time (temporality). By implication of Merleau-Ponty's idea of them being existentials, they cannot be separated from each other and each existential is embedded and interwoven with the other. Fundamental to Merleau-Ponty's theses is that the person is the body, which is the embodiment of mind and body into one. This is the opposite of the Cartesian worldview where mind and body are separate and mind takes precedent over the body. Merleau-Ponty (1989: 12) summarises this as: 'our relation to the world is not that of a thinker to an object of thought'. Further, the body inhabits space and because of this it is also within time. For Merleau-Ponty space is not an abstract entity that merely maps itself onto the body. Instead the body actively occupies space through perception, intentional movement and activity (1962: 136). Space does not exist outside the body as space is experienced from within the body. Neither does the mind map itself onto the body. Consequently, the body is not moved by the mind. Further, bodily movement can be best or only fully understood at a preconscious level because it is the body not the mind that is in space and time. Thus, in the explication of this theory, the lived body (with flesh and depth) and existential space and time must be constantly accounted for. Further, not to take account of spatiality, temporality, or the various dimensions of perception would be inadequate and would de-contextualise and de-humanise lived experience.

Merleau-Ponty's ideas on embodiment, especially in the context of people with impaired cognition such as people living with dementia, offer a radically different and even hopeful construction of the body as an agent that is trying to act appropriately based on perception, even where the brain and/or mind may be said not to be cognitively intact. This position challenges existing views of what it means to have personhood and what is required to have the social status of a person.

Stoddart (1998) suggests that embodied understandings of persons brings into place emotional and relational aspects of what it means to be human. Drawing on the work of Anderson (1982), Stoddart raises the idea of 'co-humanity' suggesting that people only become the people they are when they enter into relationship with others. We each relate to and with others, we respond to people, to circumstances and environments thus shaping and co-creating the social world. Stoddart (1998) argues that this relational existence creates personal growth that is not dependent on cognitive or reflective attributes. Stoddart draws on Niebhur's (1963) idea of the person being *'response-able'*.

> By response-ability, Niebuhr means that: (i) we respond to action upon us, (ii) our responses are the result of our interpretation of those actions, (iii) we anticipate that our responses will be met by the responses of other people (i.e. we are accountable to others), and (iv) in responding we recognise our social solidarity of continually forming society as we all respond to each other.
>
> (Stoddart, 1998: 10)

Co-humanity means that persons are not dependent on particular attributes, characteristics or cognitive processes (such as reflection) in order to be a person. Instead the personal growth that continually happens through embodied engagement with the social world shapes our continual existence as persons. Carol Gilligan (1982) suggests that we should consider each of us as existing in 'attached' relationships. For Gilligan, each person is immersed in a web of ongoing relationships and being 'in relation' to another is a fundamental part of human existence. Persons are defined by their historical connections and relationships. A moral relationship is not about how one impersonal person reacts towards another (impersonal person). Instead the essence of morality is located in the interrelationship of the subjective experiences that both individuals bring to the relationship.

The recognition of a person's history acknowledges their social, psychological and cultural biography and in acknowledging this biography, development continues through the life-span, *'forming the tapestry of one's life'* (Selder, 1989). A person's reality refers to the everyday world. It is imbued with personal meanings, beliefs and values which are essential to the way the person 'sees' themselves and the way their world is constructed. Whilst many aspects of an individual's reality may be shared with others so that common understandings can exist in order to form a sense of community, it is the individuality of our personal meanings that determines 'who I am'. It is a rich tapestry of meaning that creates the foundation on which the structures of one's life are built. When the threads of such a tapestry are severed and torn, as occurs through major life events such as illness and disability, then a once stable foundation becomes unstable and the structures of one's life fall.

Connecting Concepts of Persons through Authenticity

So far we have explored four differing but related concepts of 'person' – the attributes, reflective, moral and embodied perspectives. Each of these perspectives place a different lens on different philosophical positions and the ways in which these lenses shape our thinking about persons and ultimately the way we make decisions. However, no one position stands alone when thinking about decision-making in practice. The reality is that we may have to draw from all these perspectives in order to make informed person-centred decisions. One way of enabling such integration to happen is through the concept of 'authenticity'.

> By authentic is meant a way of reaching decisions which are truly one's own – decisions that express all that one believes important about oneself and the world, the entire complexity of one's values.
>
> (Gadow, 1980: 85)

The word 'authentic' is often used in discussions about autonomous decision-making (Kant [Sullivan, 1990]; Christman, 1989; Dworkin, 1991). Dworkin (1991), for example, argues that to be autonomous a person must have desires that can authentically be considered one's

own, with processes of socialisation in society recognised as a necessary part of developing authenticity and a unique set of values
(Meyers, 1989). An individual's life is always embedded in the culture of the communities from which identity is derived (MacIntyre,
1992). People have a past, present and future and to detach oneself
from the past serves to deform the present and plans for the future.

Heidegger (1990: 345) argues that authenticity would be completely misunderstood if it was seen to consist of simply taking up
possibilities which have been proposed and recommended, and
seizing hold of them. Being authentic requires us to consider such
factors as the meaning of individual relationships, emotional engagement, knowledge and decision-making capacity in determining our
'being in the world'. Heidegger argues that only those options that
are seen to 'belong' should be considered. This suggests though that
some things might not belong and can be discarded. Returning to
our earlier argument about the problem of rational reflection and the
mind–body split, it is important to consider the rationale for discard-
ing things and who it is that makes such decisions. The potential
is great for people with altered cognition and/or severe disabilities
to be treated as a 'thing' that can be discarded. In arguing against
us having fixed perceptions of persons and their being in the world,
Heidegger uses the analogy of equipment in a workshop. If a piece of
equipment is damaged, one option is to discard it, another option is
to alter its purpose and utility. Just because something cannot be used
for its original purpose does not mean that it is devoid of any purpose
whatsoever – *The damage to the equipment is still not a mere altera-
tion of a thing* (Heidegger, 1990: 103). Unless we continue to see
the damaged equipment as having meaning, then the equipment that
we do accord a usefulness to loses some of its meaning – *it reveals
itself as something just present-at-hand and no more, which cannot
be budged without the thing that is missing* (Heidegger, 1990: 103).
Here, the accumulative life experience that a person brings to a given
situation imbues meaning on the situation itself and current practice.
The worth of a person then, is more than an instrumental worth,
but represents the positive notion of freedom articulated by Berlin
(1992) as thinking, willing and active beings. A person's authenticity
is composed of 'signs'.

> Among signs there are symptoms, warning signals, signs of things
> that have happened already, signs by which things are recognized;
> these have different ways of indicating, regardless of what may be
> serving as such a sign.
>
> (Heidegger, 1990: 108)

'Signs' represent our lives, that is beliefs, values and life experiences.
We can treat these either as detached things that have little significance, or we can view them as being central to our lives. It is not
enough to just take note of another's beliefs, values, views and experiences. They must be integrated into the being in the world for
that individual. Being conscious of another's beliefs and values does

not provide a prescription for action, but instead provides guidance towards the most appropriate approach for action based on the individual's life experience. In recognition of this interconnectedness, the individuality of all parties is made explicit in the relationship. Such an approach requires commitment on the part of persons to want to engage in such a relationship and to accept it.

Taking note of 'signs' enables a person to place actions in context or as MacIntyre (1992: 210) suggests, *the act of utterance becomes intelligible by finding its place in a narrative*. In other words, for an individual's values to have meaning they need to be placed in the context of their lives, as we only become aware of our values when they are challenged either positively or negatively (Heidegger, 1990: 112). Without clarifying the meaning of a value in its original context, then it may be difficult to move it from something that is available to us, to something that guides action. If a value cannot be clarified, that doesn't mean it doesn't exist but other values may be needed to access it. For example, even if a person values the right to determine decisions for him/herself, it may not be possible for another person to understand the importance of that value to him/her until other values have been clarified, such as those the person holds about (for example) the importance of fairness and justice in society.

From the perspective of caring, taking note of 'signs' enables the facilitation of decision-making from the patient's perspective, that is facilitate their authenticity. Heidegger argues that when the maintenance of another's authenticity is not a priority in caring practices then there is a danger of stepping into the place of the other and solving the problems or meeting the needs on behalf of the other. Heidegger calls such *practice 'defective solicitude'*, for one becomes dominant and the other is made dependent, thus reducing the other to a thing. In a 'freedom-gaining' relationship (Barker, 1991), one looks ahead with the other to help him or her understand what lies ahead and to develop appropriate coping mechanisms. There are times when such a partnership may not be possible and that one may have to 'leap ahead' of the other in order to facilitate the other's authenticity. The goal remains that of helping the other recognise what he/she needs for him or herself and to develop a mechanism for the other to cope successfully on their own. One steps back to enable the other to deploy his or her strategies, but steps forward to support in times of weakness, leaving the other free to determine his or her own fate (Heidegger, 1990: 159; Barker, 1991: 191). This concept of authenticity concurs with philosophies of 'personhood' (Kitwood, 1997) within a nurse–patient relationship that requires involvement, risk taking, stepping back to create space and stepping forwards in times of vulnerability.

Viewing personhood as authenticity, starts from the position that everyone has 'inborn potential', but that individuals learn how to exercise that potential through socialisation. All adults have the same inborn potential but that potential is fully realized or not through processes of socialisation. Various internal and external constraints may be in place that prevent an individual's full potential from being realized and thus, people may need assistance in determining the most appropriate course of action. This approach demands that the nurse's role should focus on facilitating an individual's authenticity, so that their full potential can be realised and their capacity to exercise autonomous action maximised through facilitating the erosion of constraining factors.

The 'Life Plan' as a representation of the Authentic Self

Knowing how to maximise an individual's autonomy is a key consideration in PCN and one that will be addressed in later chapters of this book. Having some sense of what authenticity means to a person and how that manifests itself through their being-in-the-world is essential to working in a person-centred way. One way of thinking about this is through the idea of a 'life plan'.

A life plan is not merely a list of objectives with a plan and strategies for carrying them out – a mechanical list. A life plan is a presentation of what a person wants to do in life (Meyers, 1989: 49). This life plan may be written down (a biography could be seen as a representation of a life plan) or it may be a verbal articulation of life priorities, goals, ambitions, dreams and desires. A life plan enables reflection on life goals within the context of achieving integration in ones' life. Life plans evolve over time, with new experiences that are consistent with one's life plan being integrated into it in order to create future goals and projects. A life plan would include at least one activity that the person wants to pursue, or a value that the person wants to advance or an emotional bond that the person wants to sustain. As most people have a variety of activities, values and emotions that they would wish to be identified with, then typically a life plan would consist of an ordering of assorted desires and concerns and some ordering of their priority, so that they can invest time and energy appropriately:

> . . . it recognizes that the authentic self is dynamic and explains how individuals can gain control over their selves, along with their conduct. . . . The self of the person who exercises autonomy competency, then, is an authentic self – a self-chosen identity rooted in the individual's most abiding feelings and firmest convictions, yet subject to the critical perspective autonomy competency affords.
>
> (Meyers, 1989: 61)

So, for example, the older person considering the option of moving to residential care, may list values such as retention of their independence, family contact, contact with friends and colleagues, being able to attend religious services in their local church, being able to eat what they want and when they want it, as values that they hold central to their decision-making. However, maintaining contact with their family may be the overriding desire and therefore assumes greater importance than other desires. In choosing suitable residential care, this desire would be given greatest priority.

However, throughout the life-span, individuals continually grow, develop and experience transition and so there is always the potential for a new direction in life to be taken. So long as this new direction is consistent with the individual's authenticity, then the evolving-self can be accommodated. If a person's life plan contains conflicting traits and goals, then the individual can be paralysed by confusion and ambivalence and would rarely be able to act with confidence that the action satisfactorily represents his or her true self (Meyers, 1989). Reflection on the effectiveness of decisions is always considered against authenticity. In terms of making choices within a life plan, Meyers adopts Rawls (1992) perspective on rational choice. The making of choices has two components – rational choice and deliberative rationality.

For a choice to be rational, a person must know what sorts of things are important to them, must evaluate the relative intensity of their desires, must order their preferences consistently and must envisage alternative plans for action (Rawls, 1992: 418,419). These principles enable people to opt for the plan that will enable the achievement of more 'ends' than other potential plans and for the one that is most likely to succeed. Whilst Rawls argues from a rational perspective that decisions should be postponed until all necessary information has been availed of, he does also recognise that being aware of the dominant values in one's life and aiming to achieve unity and consistency of values, should enable the making of decisions based on what they intuitively know is best for them (Rawls, 1992: 412). In the making of rational choice, the principle of adopting the plan which maximises the expected net balance of satisfactions is the one to be chosen, that is, the person should choose the course that is most likely to achieve their most important aims (Rawls, 1992: 416).

Deliberative rationality is the choosing of the plan that is most consistent with one's overall values and other principles, such as, being consistent with the dominant theme in one's decisions and the avoidance of inconsistency (Rawls, 1992: 417). However, Meyers rightly argues that without others' interpretations of choices, then the process of deliberation is reduced to an individualistic self-referential process.

Life plans are formed through, memory, reflection, imagination and through conversation with others. Through reflection on an individual's values, individual traits and broad ambitions, various options for action are outlined. Evaluation of an option is undertaken based on its consistency with overall values, its potential for achieving more 'ends' than other potential plans, the one that is most likely to succeed, but most importantly, the one that is most likely to achieve their most important aims. It may be necessary to divide an option up into particular segments to enable thorough reflection and evaluation. The person can explore how they would feel about particular outcomes from choosing that option or how they would behave if that outcome was chosen. Their attraction to or aversion from the potential outcomes and behaviours and their strength of feeling about these provides a yardstick for assessment of options.

Meyers (1989: 83) argues that unless people are able to carry out their desired life plans, then their deliberations will be wasted. She suggests that both 'resistance' and 'resolve' are required to do this – resistance of unwarranted pressure from other individuals and resolve in one's determination to act on his or her own judgements. However, we know how difficult it is for many users of health and social care services to sustain their resistance and resolve in the making of authentic decisions.

Summary of Key Points

In this chapter we have presented some conceptual and philosophical perspectives on personhood and person-centredness. There is no definitive framework available to conceptualise these so we have offered one way of doing this, through four different perspectives – the attributes, reflective, moral and embodied perspectives. These are not mutually exclusive perspectives and indeed when one explores them through the unifying concept of 'authenticity' then the areas of overlap are obvious. In the real world of course we do not think about our own and others being in this fragmented way and indeed to do so would lead to faulty decision-making and the potential erosion of a person's personhood as it would create 'blind-spots' in our reflection and decision-making. However, we need to be aware of these dimensions when making decisions, as to not consider one aspect can lead to faulty decision-making in the other. Whilst authenticity can be seen to be a unifying concept in enabling more effective decision-making, we need to be acutely aware of the fact that many people are unable to represent their authentic self autonomously and so need help from others in situations where their authenticity may be under threat. Having some understanding of another's 'life plan' enables us to potentially provide such help to another person. For the majority of people, a life plan is not a written, structured document that is carried around in daily life! However, think about our closest friendships and relationships – in these relationships we share our deepest sense of 'self' with others, enabling others to know who I am as a person, what values are important to me, the dreams, hopes and desires I hold in my life and the kind of life that I strive to live. This is a life plan. Through our discussions, reflections, debates, arguments and agreements the life plan is shaped and reshaped, ordered and reordered, prioritised and reprioritized as my life progresses. Take such a dynamic into a professional relationship and as a nurse facilitating the care of another person, that life plan translates into (for example) a formal comprehensive assessment that includes a 'biographical assessment'. We will argue that 'knowing the person' in this way is essential to PCN.

Endnote

1. Tardive dyskinesia is a variety of dyskinesia (involuntary, repetitive movements) manifesting as a side effect of long-term or high-dose use of dopamine antagonists, usually antipsychotics. Tardive dyskinesia is characterised by repetitive, involuntary, purposeless movements. Features of the disorder may include grimacing, tongue protrusion, lip smacking, puckering and pursing of the lips and rapid eye blinking. Rapid movements of the extremities may also occur. Impaired movements of the fingers may also appear.

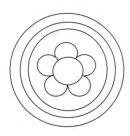

Chapter 3

A Theoretical Framework for Person-Centred Nursing

Introduction

In the previous chapter you will have had the opportunity to explore personhood, an important philosophical basis underpinning PCN. In this chapter we would like to introduce the PCN Framework, and help place this framework in the context of existing theoretical and research literature. The origins of the Framework draw on original work focusing on caring in nursing as perceived by patients and nurses (McCance, 2003), and person-centred practice with older people (McCormack, 2001b). The concepts of caring and person-centredness will be explored in more detail in an attempt to demonstrate: (1) their relevance to nursing; (2) the synergy between the two concepts and (3) how this relates to the development of the PCN Framework.

Caring and Person-Centredness

There is a drive to redress the imbalance in care from an ethos that is medically dominated, disease orientated and often fragmented, to one that is relationship focused, collaborative and holistic. The challenges, however, in making the shift to a more holistic model of care are continually emphasised, and at one level we can attribute this to the complexity of healthcare systems and the impact of a diverse range of strategy and policy imperatives (Turner-Stokes, 2007). This inevitably translates into challenges experienced at practice level that include, for example:

- increase emphasis on targets
- the impact of organisational culture on individuals and teams

- the increase in treatment options and technological care
- the requirement of professionals to be technically competent
- the drive for effectiveness and efficiency and an unrelenting focus on the financial bottom line

There is currently, however, within the United Kingdom, an increasing desire to reaffirm the importance of the fundamentals of care, such as dignity, respect, privacy and communication (DoH, 2006; DHSSPS, 2008; RCN, 2008), which are considered important to the patient. (Chapter 1 provides a more detailed analysis of the policy context and how this relates to the development of person-centred practice.) It is in this context that we find increasing attention being given to therapeutic caring and person-centred practice, approaches that place the human experience at the centre of care delivery. There is a strong synergy between caring and person-centredness, with both ultimately about the development of therapeutic relationships (McCormack & McCance, 2006). It is clear, however, that whilst both terms are synergistic they are not synonymous, with differences evident in how they have been defined in the literature, and in relation to conceptual and theoretical developments. Each of these areas will be considered in turn.

The Concept of Caring

The concept of caring has been the subject of much debate in relation to definition and meaning. This debate has been ongoing since the 1970s when caring was a concept considered to be synonymous with nursing (McFarlane, 1976; Leininger, 1981), yet a concise definition has not been established. In fact the international literature is peppered with many concept analyses of caring, all making the same claim that a concise definition of caring within nursing still remains elusive (e.g. Wilkinson, 1998; McCance et al., 1999; Lin & Chiou, 2003; Brilowski & Wendler, 2005). This subsequently provides the necessary justification for the proliferation of research studies, which attempt to explore the experience of caring, with a view to providing greater understanding of the concept, several of which will be referred to throughout this and other chapters. It is not the purpose within this chapter to analyse all that has been published to date on the concept of caring, nor indeed to suggest our own definition of caring, but rather to provide a general understanding of the concept in light of the evidence. In an attempt to do this we would like to draw on the seminal work of Morse et al. (1991), who conducted one of the early concept analysis on caring. Within this seminal work 35 authors' definitions of caring were considered and the main characteristics of their perspective identified. Content analysis revealed five perspectives on caring: caring as a human trait; caring as a moral imperative; caring as an affect, caring as an interpersonal interaction; and caring as a therapeutic intervention. Each of these perspectives illustrates the complexity of caring as a concept, and still have resonance for nursing today.

Caring as a human trait

Caring as a human trait, according to Morse et al. (1991), describes caring as 'a universal characteristic . . . that forms the foundation of human society' and is 'necessary for human survival – an essential component of being human' (p.122). Existential philosophers such as Heidegger (1962), Sartre (1972) and Buber (1958) have contributed to this perspective, presenting the notion that care is a way of being in the world, that is, to care is to be human. The early writings of Martin Heidegger is the philosophy most frequently cited by nurses in relation to caring (Brykczynska, 1997). Molina (1962) comments that Heidegger's choice of the word care to describe the total structure of the person is to emphasise the intimacy of the relationship between the person and the world. Furthermore, Heidegger (1962) distinguishes between authentic and inauthentic being, and Warnock (1970), when commenting on Heidegger's work, highlighted that authentic existence can only begin when we have truly understood what we are: 'that human reality is characterised by the fact that each human being is, uniquely, himself and no-one else, and that each of us has his own possibilities to fulfil' (p. 55). This idea is central to the concept of personhood, which has been discussed in detail in Chapter 2.

Roach (1984), in her monograph on caring in nursing similarly presents the stance that caring is the human mode of being, which she has interpreted in the light of Heidegger's work. As a result, she believes that nursing is the 'professionalisation of human caring through deliberate affirmation of caring as the human mode of being' (p. 1). Benner and Wrubel (1989) also view caring as that which 'sets up a world and creates meaningful distinctions' (p. 1). It is caring which is 'essential if the person is to live in a differentiated world where some things really matter, whilst others are less important or not important at all' (p. 1). Furthermore, philosophers such as Mayeroff (1971) and Gaylin (1979) are of the opinion that caring is essential to human growth and development. This opinion is shared by Leininger (1981) and Watson (1979), two of the most prominent nursing theorists on caring. Brykczynska (1997) comments that advocates of Heideggarian ontology interpret caring in nursing terms as follows:

> They see nursing as locating its being, that is, its essence, in the practice of caring. Caring they claim gives nursing its heart and soul. Without caring, nursing is but a collection of highly skilled tasks and endeavours – a recognizable body but without an animated soul (p. 4).

Caring as a moral imperative

Within caring there is a philosophy of moral commitment that reflects a fundamental respect for preserving humanity. This is the perspective reflected by Morse et al. (1991) when they describe caring as a moral imperative that is concerned with 'maintaining the dignity and respect of patients as *people*' (p. 123). In this context, several authors have described caring as an ethic (Carper, 1978; Kelly, 1988; Fry, 1989; Harrison, 1990). For example, Watson (1985) describes caring as the moral ideal of nursing, translated as that which 'has to become a will, an intention, or commitment, that manifests itself in concrete acts' (p. 32). Similarly, Roach (1984) includes conscience, a state of moral awareness, as one of the five Cs of human caring, and Gadow (1985) describes caring within the nurse–patient relationship as a moral ideal which 'entails a commitment to a particular end' (p. 32).

Implicit in this perspective is 'respect for persons' which has also been discussed as a basis for caring (Gaut, 1983; Gadow, 1985; Kitson, 1987). Gaut (1983) specified respect for persons as one of the essential conditions of caring: 'the notion of "respect for persons" is crucial to the discussion of caring, for it entails an attitude necessary in the carer' (p. 320). Jameton (1984) discusses the concept of respect for persons in relation to two principles: (1) people should be treated with empathetic consideration; and (2) people should not be treated as a mere means to an end. The first principle includes 'listening to others, understanding them, and responding with appreciation of their intentions' (Jameton, 1984: 125). This focuses on the attitude portrayed by the manner in which the professional interacts with an individual. The second principle refers to respect for autonomy, which involves the realisation that the person has an autonomous nature, is self-determining and self-governing (Downie & Calman, 1994). According to Beauchamp and Walters (1989), 'to respect the autonomy of such self-determining agents is to recognise them as entitled to determine their own destiny, with due regard to their considered evaluations and view of the world' (p. 29). This is reflected in Gaut's (1983) analysis on caring, where respect for persons is considered 'a principle or norm for action that also must include respect for that person's actions, decisions, values and claims' (p. 319). This description of caring places it right at the heart of personhood.

Caring as an interpersonal interaction

This perspective focuses attention on the interaction between the nurse and the patient, which encompasses both the feelings and behaviours occurring within that relationship. The interpersonal dimension of caring has been confirmed more recently by Finfgeld-Connett (2008) who undertook an analysis of the concept using meta-synthesis methods. The findings from the synthesis of 49 qualitative studies and 6 concept analyses described caring as 'a context-specific interpersonal process that is characterised by expert nursing practice, interpersonal sensitivity and intimate relationships' (p. 196). She describes interpersonal sensitivity, one of the attributes of the caring process, as going beyond the routine, demonstrated through simple gestures such as attentive listening, making eye contact, touching and offering verbal reassurance.

Furthermore, the description of caring as an interpersonal interaction builds on the existential ideas that caring is part of being
human, in that existence is not only being in the world, but also
being with others in the world. Reflected in the writings of a number
of these philosophers is the idea of two general ways in which we
relate to others. In Buber's (1958) work *'I and Thou'*, a distinction is made between 'I–Thou' as that which is spoken with the
whole being, and 'I–It' as that which can never be spoken with the
whole being. When we don't relate to another person, but turn
him into an object, we are relating in the 'I–It'. When attempting
to understand the world of relation, Marcel (1981) in his study of
the 'interpersonal' discusses the idea of availability, which expresses
the willingness to put oneself at the disposal of others. According
to Marcel, it is this kind of availability which enables a person to
be present with the other, denoting presence as something rather
different and more comprehensive than being physically present.
The notion of being 'authentically' present has been discussed by
some nurse theorists (Roach, 1984; Paterson & Zderad, 1988;
Benner & Wrubel, 1989) and will be discussed in greater detail in
Chapter 6.

Caring as an affect

From this perspective caring is described as 'an emotion, as a feeling
of compassion or empathy for the patient which motivates the nurse
to provide care for the patient' (Morse et al., 1991: 123). *Caring
as an affect* emphasises the nature of the emotional involvement in
caring. This reflects the 'care about' dimension which relates to the
idea of caring as emotional attachment or affection as opposed to
the 'care for' dimension, which describes the act of caring as providing some sort of service. Jecker and Self (1991) in an analysis
of historical and contemporary images of nursing and medicine also
recognised the two senses of caring as 'caring for' and 'caring about'.
This dichotomy has also been alluded to by other authors, for example, Woodward (1997) discusses instrumental caring as that which
involves actions (care for), and expressive caring as that which 'makes
a qualitative difference in the way in which activities are undertaken'
(p. 1000) (care about). The 'care about' dimension is reflected in the
early work of Stevens-Barnum (1994) who viewed this as emotional
investment in the patients' welfare and indicates an attitudinal or
emotional dimension. Gaut (1983) and Griffin (1983) also identify
caring as a form of emotional involvement, for example, fondness,
liking for someone, attachment. This is suggestive of the notion of
caring as a form of loving, which was the conclusion from Ray's
(1981) philosophical analysis. This has been a focus for further
discussion within the literature (Campbell, 1984; Jacono, 1993),
but is an idea that can be difficult to comprehend in the context of
professional nursing.

Caring as a therapeutic intervention

Caring as a therapeutic intervention focuses on caring actions that respond to patient need that should result in positive improvements. The description of an intervention as therapeutic is suggestive of positive outcomes for the patient as a result of caring. This is reflected in the recent meta-analysis undertaken by Finfgeld-Connett (2007) who identified outcomes for both the patient and the nurse. For the patient, this is described as physical and mental well-being and is comparable to McCance's (2003) findings, which are reflected in her conceptual framework for caring in nursing. Mental well-being is considered the main outcome for the nurse, which could be translated through constructs such as decreased job-related stress and increased job satisfaction (Slater, McCormack & Bunting, 2009). Outcomes relating to the PCN Framework will be discussed in detail in Chapter 7.

Points to Ponder

Caring has a long association with nursing. What relevance do you believe the concept of caring has to everyday nursing practice?

The Concept of Person-Centredness

The terminology relating to person-centredness, whilst the subject of less intense debate, has also been discussed in the literature. Person-centred, patient-centred, client-centred and individualised care are examples of terms often used interchangeably to express the idea of person-centredness (Slater, 2006; Leplege et al., 2007). At the risk of complicating matters further, Nolan and colleagues have also introduced the concept of relationship-centred care, arguing for a move away from what they perceive as a focus on meeting individual needs, to focusing on interactions among all parties involved in care whose needs should be taken account of if good care is to result (Nolan et al., 2004). Several analyses have been conducted in an attempt to define core attributes of person-centredness, although this activity is only a relatively recent development in the contemporary literature (McCormack, 2004; Slater, 2006; Leplege et al., 2007). An early definition of person-centredness, however, is provided by Kitwood (1997), and continues to be widely used. He describes person-centredness as '. . . a standing or status that is bestowed upon one human being by others, in the context of relationship and social being. It implies recognition, respect and trust.' (p. 8). Based on an extensive review of the literature, and using the definition provided by Kitwood, McCormack (2004) argues that there are four core concepts at the heart of PCN: being in relation, being in a social world, being in place and being with self. Table 3.1 describes the links made by McCormack (2004) between the four core concepts

Table 3.1 Relationship between Kitwood's definition and concepts of person-centredness

Concept	Link with Kitwood's definition
Being in relation	Persons exist in relationships with other persons
Being in a social world	Persons are social being
Being in place	Persons have a context through which their personhood is articulated
Being with self	Being recognised, respected and trusted as a person impacts on a persons' sense of self

(Reprinted from McCormack, 2004: 33)

derived from the literature and the components of Kitwood's definition. These four core concepts will be used as a basis for discussing the meaning and enhancing understanding of person-centredness as a concept, supported by the use of stories, poetry and images.

Being in relation

Being in relation emphasises the importance of relationships and the interpersonal processes that enable the development of relationships that have therapeutic benefit. Indeed, models of nursing, irrespective of their philosophical underpinnings have emphasised the importance of relationships (e.g. Peplau, 1952; Watson, 1985; Rogers, 1980; Boykin & Schoenhofer, 1993). Recent critiques in the gerontology literature, however, argue that the term 'person-centred' fails to recognise the importance of relationships. Nolan et al. (2001) argues that person-centredness focuses (in the care literature) on the primacy of the personhood of the person being cared for, at the expense of those doing the caring, and conclude that in gerontology, the term 'relationship-centred care' is more appropriate. Whilst one can never dispute the importance of relationships in person-centredness, one can see from Kitwood's definition that 'relationship' is only one component of personhood. In PCN, the relationship between the nurses and the person being cared for is paramount. Furthermore, it has been argued that sustaining a relationship that is nurturing to both nurse and patient, requires valuing of self, moral integrity, reflective ability, knowing of self and others and flexibility derived from reflection on values and their place in the relationship (Evans, 1996; Nolan, 2001; Nolan et al., 2001; Dewing 2002; McCormack, 2003; Packer, 2003; Titchen & McGinley, 2003). Being in relation is also reflected in one of seven attributes of person-centredness identified by Slater's (2006) concept analysis – evidence of a therapeutic relationship between person and healthcare provider. Slater (2006) describes this as a partnership between the person and carer that ensures the person's own decisions are valued, in a relationship that is based on mutual trust, mutuality, is non-judgemental and does not focus on the balance of power.

I (Sally) have been working with the social services to find a suitable place for my mother (Olivia) for respite care. Mother has early onset Alzheimer's disease and whilst she continues to be able to do most things for herself, her memory is rapidly deteriorating. I am married to Noel and together we organise a rota of visits to her throughout the week to ensure her personal safety. Social services are also wonderful and they provide mother with her daily personal care and meals services. However, Noel and I need a break and want to have a holiday away for a couple of weeks, and this is my dilemma. Despite needing a break, I don't want to leave mother alone and equally don't want to place her in residential care even if it is only for a couple of weeks. You see, I know mother and all her foibles and little ways. I have spent a long time with the carers ensuring that they know these also. By working with the carers that come in each day to mother, I have helped them to get to know her very well and they seem to engage in a way that even I struggle with at times – but then they don't have all the 'mother–daughter baggage' to contend with. One carer in particular (Helen) seems to have a deep personal relationship with mother and the way that she trusts Helen is amazing. She works with mother in a way that is so tolerant and seems to forgive her overpowering ways and sense that she is 'always right' (even when she is not!). Helen never judges her and works with her to find solutions. In many ways I have learned a lot from watching Helen and oddly, I think it has helped my relationship with mother too. Helen has offered to take mother to the care home that we seem to be agreeing would be the home of choice for her respite care and help her to get a 'sense and feel of the place'. Mother is excited by this, but I'm worried – not sure what it is that I am worried about, but probably I am aware that my relationship with mother is changing and we are in a state of transition with this. Who knows how it will end up and Noel is convinced that it will all work out. I know that we will be okay, that Helen will help us through this and that we will nurture each other as we change and grow together.

Being in a social context

Earlier it was outlined how Merleau-Ponty considers persons to be interconnected with their social world, creating and recreating meaning through their being in the world. In terms of being authentic then, it was also suggested that 'signs' are significant representations of what is important in our lives. Signs are best represented through our values and our values are articulated through biography (i.e. who we are as a person). There is an increasing literature in gerontology on the value of biography (see e.g. Kenyon et al., 2001 for an edited volume of studies in narrative gerontology). Biographical approaches are not just about 'collecting stories' as a part of assessment. Instead, respect for the older person's narrative reflects the Kantian ideal of respect for the intrinsic worth of a person (Ford & McCormack, 2000; Wright & McCormack, 2001). These narratives afford the opportunity to understand the older person's context.

Meyers (1989) makes a convincing argument for the use of 'life plans' in gerontology in order to truly understand a person's context and these have been explored in some detail in Chapter 2. Applying the principle of 'life-plans' should be no different for those patients being cared for in, for example, an acute hospital setting than it is for people in residential/continuing care. The emphasis should still be on an accurate assessment of what is important to each patient and in that context being able to understanding the potential impact of their hospital stay. The ability to work with patients' beliefs and values will be discussed in more detail in Chapter 6.

Aidan is 28 and a keen motorcyclist. Recently Aidan had a biking accident resulting in a serious head injury. Whilst in the acute care setting, the care team interviewed his wife (Roisin), his dad (Frank) and his mum (Carol) as part of his assessment process. The team in the acute unit work on the principle that having a complete as possible picture of the person in a social context is vital to their recovery. Roisin, Frank and Carol completed a life-story book that was placed alongside his physical and psychological assessment. The staff used the life story to identify key aspects of Aidan's care that should be prioritised as an early part of his rehabilitation. Aidan made a good recovery but needed to spend some time in the Regional Brain Injury Unit for further rehabilitation. His life-story book played a significant role in ensuring a seamless transfer of care from the acute setting to the rehabilitation unit. His family felt very much in control of what was happening and felt they were able to guide care decisions (when Aidan was unable) in ways that they knew Aidan would approve of.

Being in place

Andrews (2003) argues that the concept of 'place' and its impact on care experiences is poorly understood in nursing. Few studies have been undertaken to assess the impact of place on patients' experiences. Dementia care mapping has been well developed in dementia care (Kitwood, 1997; Younger & Martin, 2000; Martin & Younger, 2001; Brooker, 2002; Wylie et al., 2002) and it represents one of the only assessment and care planning approaches in gerontology that formally recognises the impact of the 'milieu of care' on the care experience. Paying attention to 'place' in care relationships is increasingly recognised as important (Hussain & Raczka, 1997; Luckhurst & Ray, 1999; Andrews, 2003). When facilitating person-centredness nurses find they not only balance competing care values, but often they find it necessary to also consider organisational values (Woods, 2001). Nurses are not free to fulfil a moral obligation to the patient without considering organisational and professional implications (Johns, 1995). Whilst the freedom of the nurse is a significant issue in the facilitation of person-centredness, other characteristics of context have been found to be of equal significance, such as systems of decision-making, staff relationships, organisational systems, power differentials and the potential of the organisation to tolerate innovate practices and risk-taking. These findings have been supported in a recent analysis of the concept of context (McCormack et al., 2002). There is also evidence to suggest that the care environment has the greatest potential to enhance or limit the facilitation of person-centred practice (Tonuma & Wimbolt, 2000; McCormack, 2001a).

Sensing, Feeling, Belonging

Sunshine on my face where are you?
Rain falling through my fingers where are you?
Wind in my hair where are you?
Frost chapping my lips where are you?

Childhood memories a distant
Of running through fresh-mown hay
Smelling the softness of summer
Tasting the joy of nature's abundance

Owning the spaces in my soul
Longing for the places that renew
Seeking connection with loves joys
Knowing my losses are life's gains

Bathing in the streams of youthful abundance
Restricted smells of care and kindness
Replacing with memories of loving and being loved
Embraced in sexual exuberance forgotten

Sunshine on my face I need you
Rain falling through my fingers I want you
Wind in my hair deserted me?
Frost chapping my lips never more

(Anonymous)

Being with self

Respect for values is central to person-centred practice (Williams & Tappen, 1999; Clarke, 2000; McCormack, 2001b) and places a responsibility on the nurse to develop a clear picture of what the patient values about their life and how they make sense of what is happening to them (Brown et al., 1997). This provides a standard against which the nurse can compare current decisions and behaviours of the patient with those values and preferences made in life in general, and which form the basis of a life plan (Meyers, 1989). Assisting the individual to find meaning in care, may help them to tolerate the incongruity of their current situation in relation to their goals for the future. This reflects the stance of the philosopher John McMurray (1995), who argues for the primacy of 'self as agent', emphasising the importance of the person 'knowing self' through values clarification. This, however, is not just applicable to the patient in the care situation, but also applies to nurses involved in care delivery who need to be aware of 'self' and how their own values and beliefs can impact on decisions made about a patient's care and treatment – something that is addressed further in Chapter 4. This reinforces the centrality of shared decision-making in healthcare and the need for a 'negotiated' approach between practitioner and patient.

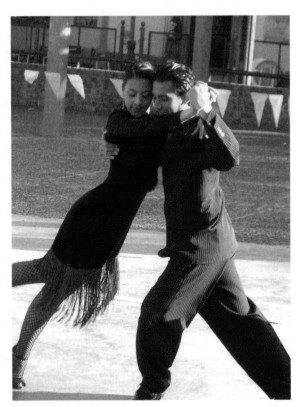

"So partnership working, whether you're an equal partner or seen as a junior partner it's a relationship – bottom line: sharing views, and sharing experience and working together to improve something that's beyond both partners, both sharing a mutual interest. It's like a dance – a tango between friends" (Comment from participant in the Republic of Ireland Older Persons National Practice Development Programme, McCormack et al 2009c)

Person-Centred Nursing

Complementarity between the concept of caring and the concept of person-centredness is evident on a number of levels:

- they reflect the tenets of existential philosophy
- theoretically they reflect the ideals of humanistic caring
- they have a moral component
- they assume practice is based on a therapeutic intent
- they are translated in practice through relationships that are build upon effective interpersonal processes.

Furthermore, the nursing literature is consistent in the view that being person-centred requires the formation of therapeutic relationships between professionals, patients and others significant to them in their lives and that these relationships are built on mutual trust, understanding and a sharing of collective knowledge (Binnie & Titchen, 1999; McCormack, 2001a, 2004; Dewing, 2004; Nolan et al., 2004). A recent definition of person-centredness developed in a National Action Research Programme in Ireland closely reflects this literature and is consistent with the understandings of person-centredness within a nursing context.

> Person-centeredness is an approach to practice established through the formation and fostering of therapeutic relationships between all care providers, older people and others significant to them in their lives. It is underpinned by values of respect for persons, individual

right to self determination, mutual respect and understanding. It is enabled by cultures of empowerment that foster continuous approaches to practice development.

(McCormack et al., 2008b: 1)

Moving these conceptual ideas into frameworks that can be applied and evaluated in practice, however, remains the challenge. Whilst there is increased understanding of person-centredness and other related concepts that underpin nursing, how they are operationalised in practice needs to be understood if improvements in care are to be realised. Several frameworks have been developed within nursing with an explicit focus on developing person-centred practice. Examples include: the Burford NDU Model, developed with a focus on acute hospital care (Johns, 1994); the Senses Framework developed originally in the context of older people in a care home setting (Nolan et al., 2004); and the Tidal Model developed for use within mental health (Barker, 2001, 2002). The Framework described in this book, however, recognises and builds on the interconnectedness between caring and person-centredness. We would argue that the attributes of caring are implicit within a philosophy of PCN and by drawing on the existing evidence base in relation to these and other related concepts, provides a firm foundation on which to develop practice.

The Person-Centred Nursing Framework[1]

The PCN Framework was developed for use in the intervention stage of a large quasi-experimental project that focused on measuring the effectiveness of the implementation of PCN in a tertiary hospital setting (McCormack & McCance, 2006; McCormack et al., 2007). The Framework was derived from McCormack's conceptual framework (2001b, 2003) focusing on person-centred practice with older people, and McCance et al.'s framework (2001) focusing on patients and nurses experience of caring in nursing. These two conceptual frameworks were selected for the following reasons:

- they were each derived from a humanistic perspective of caring
- initial review of the frameworks indicated a high degree of consistency across individual concepts and thus a high degree of face validity
- they were both derived from inductive and systematic collaborative research processes
- collectively, they represented a synthesis of the then available literature on caring and person-centredness.

McCance et al. (2001) conducted a phenomenological study using narrative methods to explore patients' and nurses' experience of caring in nursing. The conceptual framework that emerged comprised three major constructs adapted from Donabedian's (1982) structure, process and outcome model, not unlike the approach used by Mitchell et al. (1998) to develop the 'Quality Health Outcomes Model'. Structures were categorised as: nurse attributes (professional competence, interpersonal skills, commitment to the job and personal characteristics); organisational issues (time, skill mix and the nurse's role) and patient attributes. The processes of care covered a wide range of nursing activities that constituted caring as perceived by patients and included: providing for patients' physical needs; providing for patients' psychological needs (providing information, providing reassurance, showing concern, communicating); being attentive, getting to know the patient, taking time, being firm, showing respect and the extra touch. The outcomes emanated from the process of caring and included a feeling of well-being (affective and physical), patient satisfaction and effect on the environment.

McCormack (2001b) conducted a hermeneutic study combining methods of conversation analysis in order to explore the meaning of autonomy for older people in acute care settings. Through the analysis of 14 case studies of nurse–patient relationships a conceptual framework for person-centred practice was developed based on an understanding of autonomy as 'authentic consciousness' (McCormack, 2003). The emerging conceptual framework for person-centred practice has three constructs. The first construct identified five nursing roles, referred to in the Framework as 'imperfect duties' (negotiation, informed flexibility, mutuality, transparency and sympathetic presence). The second construct articulated differing levels of engagement between patients and nurses in order to sustain a therapeutic caring relationship (engagement, partial disengagement, complete disengagement). The third construct described those factors that impact on the quality of the engagement between nurses and patients, including the context of the care environment, the nurse's values history, the patient's values history and the nurse's knowledge and experience.

Reflecting on the relationship between humanistic nursing and the concept of caring and person-centredness as discussed earlier, it is not surprising that there were commonalities between the work of McCance (2003) and McCormack (2003). Work was undertaken to develop a combined framework, with the ultimate aim of providing a mid-range theory for PCN. The origins of the Framework, with its foundations in nursing practice, provide a unique perspective for nursing that conceptually links caring and person-centredness.

Developing the Framework

The process of developing the PCN Framework, presented in Figure 3.1, involved a series of systematic steps. Identifying the similarities and matched elements of each conceptual framework was an important first step and confirmed the strong relationship between caring and person-centred practice. For example, McCormack

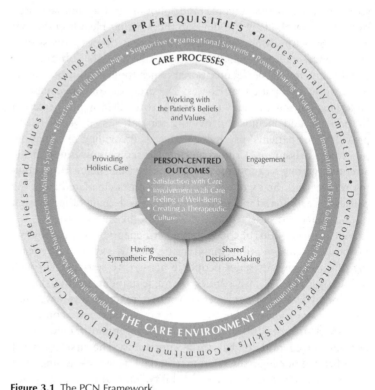

Figure 3.1 The PCN Framework.

(2003) identified contextual factors that reflected many comparable elements captured by McCance (2003) under 'structures'. Similarly, the 'imperfect duties' described by McCormack (2003) incorporated elements of the process of caring described by McCance (2003). The second step involved the exploration of areas of difference using a critical dialogue with co-researchers (*n* = 6) and with lead practitioners from a range of clinical settings (*n* = 16) as a means of reaching agreement in relation to where these elements might fit within the new framework. The concepts underpinning both conceptual frameworks were then discussed. These conversations took the form of focused discussions using critical questioning techniques to unravel each concept. The original sources of literature and data were consulted in order to ensure shared clarity of meaning of key terms in each framework. These conversations were tape-recorded and listened to after each discussion in order to identify key elements of each framework that needed to be retained or amended in the combined framework. Key concepts from both conceptual frameworks were listed and a first draft of the PCN Framework was constructed.

A period of testing the Framework was undertaken. Two focus groups were held – one with co-researchers (*n* = 6) and one with lead practitioners from a range of clinical settings (*n* = 16). The draft framework was presented and their views on clarity, coherence and comprehensibility sought. Prior to the focus groups, the individual frameworks (McCance, 2003; McCormack, 2003) were provided as background to enable discussion. Significantly, the ease with which lead practitioners engaged with the Framework and were able to contextualise elements within their clinical environments was the most important indicator. Furthermore, co-researchers were able to identify ways in which the Framework could be used in their research to focus decision-making. For example, the Framework was used to facilitate teams to analyse barriers to change (arising, for example, from differences in beliefs and values), focus particular developments in practice (e.g. the sharing of 'power' with patients) or evaluate developments as they progressed through the intervention (e.g. changes made to the care environment). The Framework has been refined with co-researchers and project participants throughout the intervention period of the larger quasi-experimental project referred to earlier.

Before describing the Framework in more detail, however, it is important to place it on the continuum of theory development, as this often influences its use in practice. In order to do this we will refer to the seminal work of Fawcett (1995), who describes a hierarchy of nursing knowledge that has five components.

At the highest level of abstraction is the meta-paradigm that represents a broad consensus for nursing, which provides general parameters for the field, and next to this are philosophies, which provide a statement of beliefs and values. Conceptual models are at the next level and provide a particular frame of reference that says something about 'how to observe and interpret the phenomena of interest to the discipline' (Fawcett, 1995: 3). Theories are the third component in the hierarchy, which are less abstract than conceptual models. They can be further described as grand theories or middle-range theories with the latter being narrower in scope and 'made up of concepts and propositions that are empirically measurable' (p. 25). Fawcett (1995) distinguishes between conceptual models and mid-range theories, in that mid-range theories articulate one or more relatively concrete and specific concepts that are derived from a conceptual model. Furthermore, the propositions that describe these concepts propose specific relationships between them. The final component in the hierarchy of nursing knowledge is empirical indicators, which provide the means of measuring concepts within a middle-range theory. The PCN Framework has been described as a middle-range theory in that it has been derived from two abstract conceptual frameworks, comprises concepts that are relatively specific, and outlines relationships between the constructs (McCormack & McCance, 2006). The following sections will describe the concepts within the Framework and how they relate, thus demonstrating its value as a middle-range theory.

Overview of the Framework

Within this section we will provide an overview of the PCN Framework and the relevance of the Framework to practice. The Framework essentially comprises four constructs:

- *prerequisites* which focus on the attributes of the nurse
- *the care environment* which focuses on the context in which care is delivered
- *person-centred processes* which focus on delivering care through a range of activities
- *expected outcomes* which are the results of effective PCN.

The relationship between the constructs of the Framework is indicated by the pictorial representation, that is, to reach the centre of the Framework, the prerequisites must first be considered, then the care environment, which are necessary in providing effective care through the care processes. This ordering, ultimately leads to the achievement of the outcomes – the central component of the Framework. It is also acknowledged that there are relationships within, and across constructs, some of which are currently being tested through further research.

The ***prerequisites*** focus on the attributes of the nurse and include: being professionally competent; having developed interpersonal skills; being committed to the job; being able to demonstrate clarity of beliefs and values; and knowing self. Professional competence focuses on the knowledge and skills of the nurse to make decisions and prioritise care, and includes competence in relation to physical or technical aspects of care. Having highly developed interpersonal skills reflects the ability of the nurse to communicate at a variety of levels. Commitment to the job is indicative of dedication and a sense that the nurse wants to provide care that is best for the patient. Clarity of beliefs and values highlights the importance of the nurse knowing his/her own views and being aware of how these can impact on decisions made by the patient. This is closely linked to knowing self and the assumption that before we can help others we need to have insight into how we function as a person.

The ***care environment*** focuses on the context in which care is delivered and includes: appropriate skill mix; systems that facilitate shared decision-making; the sharing of power; effective staff relationships; organisational systems that are supportive; the potential for innovation and risk-taking; and the physical environment. Appropriate skill mix highlights the potential impact of staffing levels on the delivery of effective person-centred care, and emphasises the importance of the composition of the team in achieving positive outcomes for patients. Shared decision-making is dependent on systems and processes being in place that facilitate a dialogue between those involved in the caring interaction. This can include patient, family member and/or carer or indeed nurse, doctor or another health professional. This is also closely linked to the development of effective staff relationships and to the sharing of power. It is, however, important to note that the sharing of power also relates to the power base between the patient and the nurse, which reflects one of the basic tenants of person-centredness described earlier. The identification of supportive organisational systems acknowledges the incredible influence organisational culture can have on the quality of care delivered and the freedom afforded to practitioners to work autonomously, reflecting the potential for innovation and risk-taking. Finally, the physical environment recognises the impact of the physical surroundings on nursing practice. These characteristics of the care environment are consistent with the conceptual development of the concept of context undertaken by McCormack et al. (2002) and Rycroft-Malone et al. (2002). Key characteristics of context arising from these studies include the culture of the workplace, the quality of nursing leadership and the commitment of the organisation to the use of multiple sources of evidence to evaluate the quality of care delivery. As previously highlighted, the care environment and the components described here have a significant impact on the operationalisation of PCN and have the greatest potential to limit or enhance the facilitation of person-centred processes (McCormack, 2004).

Person-centred processes focus on delivering care through a range of activities that operationalise PCN and include: working with patient's beliefs and values; engagement; having sympathetic presence; sharing decision-making and providing holistic care. This is the component of the Framework that specifically focuses on the patient, describing PCN in the context of care delivery. Working with patients' beliefs and values reinforces one of the fundamental principles of PCN, which places importance on developing a clear picture of what the patient values about his/her life and how he/she makes sense of what is happening. This is closely linked to shared decision-making. This focuses on nurses facilitating patient participation through providing information and integrating newly formed perspectives into established practices, but is dependent on systems that facilitate shared decision-making (the care environment). This must involve a process of negotiation that takes account of individual values to form a legitimate basis for decision-making, the success of which rests on successful processes of communication. McCormack (2004) illustrates the links between these processes stating that 'knowing what is important forms a foundation for decision-making that adopts a "negotiated" approach between practitioner and patient' (p. 35). Having sympathetic presence highlights an engagement that recognises the uniqueness and value of the individual and reflects the quality of the nurse–patient relationship. Finally, providing holistic care focuses on meeting the needs of patients, which maybe physically, psychological, social or spiritual in nature.

Outcomes are the results expected from effective PCN and include: satisfaction with care; involvement in care; feeling of wellbeing and creating a therapeutic environment. Patient satisfaction reflects the evaluation a patient places on their care experience and is arguably the most tangible outcome measure, which is well documented in the literature as an indicator of quality care (Edwards & Staniszewska, 2000; Edwards et al., 2004). Involvement in care is the outcome expected as a result of participating in shared decision-making processes. A feeling of well-being was clearly highlighted by McCance (2003) and is indicative of the patient feeling valued. Enhanced mental well-being and improvements in patients' physical well-being was similarly identified in the meta-synthesis of caring in nursing undertaken by Finfgeld-Connett (2008). Creating a therapeutic environment, described as one in which decision-making is shared, staff relationships are collaborative, leadership is transformational and innovative practices are supported, is the ultimate outcome for teams striving to develop person-centred cultures in the workplace. Identifying outcomes from effective person-centred care that are measurable, however, remains a challenge. This was an essential aspect of the research study in which this Framework was being tested, and tools have been identified from the literature and some further developed to facilitate outcome measurement (see Chapter 7).

Chapters 4–7 will explore each of the constructs within the Framework in greater detail and will use a variety of media such as stories, literary works and art to enhance understanding for the reader. The development of the PCN Framework is rooted in practice and continues to be tested on an international stage with a wide range of professional groups from different settings. It is only through using the Framework with practitioners that the validity of the constructs can be tested and further refined. This activity has taken many forms and includes use of the Framework: to facilitate reflection; as a framework for analysis of data; to guide developments in practice and to gain feedback on the user experience. Chapter 8 will draw on several international projects currently ongoing that are using the Framework in a range of different ways, to illustrate the utility and flexibility of its use in practice.

Points to Ponder

What elements of the PCN Framework can you best relate to, in everyday practice? Can you recall an event that for you represents PCN and what does the Framework tell you about that event?

Summary of Key Points

Caring and person-centredness are important concepts for nursing practice, and whilst the evidence base underpinning each differs in focus, there is a high degree of synergy between both concepts. The origins of the PCN Framework demonstrates this synergy and it has been argued in this chapter that the attributes of caring are implicit within a philosophy of PCN. The Framework highlights the complexity of PCN, and through the articulation of the key constructs, emphasises the contextual, attitudinal and moral dimensions of humanistic caring practices. The relationship between the constructs describes the necessity for competent nurses, who have the ability to manage the numerous contextual and attitudinal factors that exist within care environments, to engage in processes that keep the person at the centre of caring interactions. The dialogue created between nurses and patients illustrate the potential of PCN and the opportunity to deliver on important outcomes.

Endnote

1. The text in the remainder of this chapter is based on the original publication by McCormack & McCance (2006).

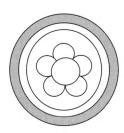

Chapter 4

Pre-requisites: Attributes of the Nurse

Introduction

In this chapter we will explore pre-requisites, the first construct within the PCN Framework, which describes the attributes of the nurse. It is important at the outset to justify the use of the term pre-requisites, which according to a standard dictionary definition implies something that is 'required or necessary as a prior condition' (www.dictionary.com). This is accurate in the context of the Framework and makes explicit the assumption that specific attributes need to be in place before a nurse is able to deliver effective person-centred care. The caring literature has a significant contribution to make in articulating qualities of the nurse that are perceived as caring, or indeed non-caring, by patients and this evidence base will be drawn on throughout the discussion. Within the Framework, five pre-requisites are identified, which are considered the essential building blocks to the delivery of person-centred care. These five attributes are presented in Figure 4.1 and will be used to shape the structure of the chapter.

Professionally Competent

Within the PCN Framework, being professionally competent is defined as 'the knowledge and skills of the nurse to make decisions and prioritise care, and includes competence in relation to physical or technical aspects of care' (McCormack & McCance, 2006: 475). At this point it is useful to articulate what we mean by the term competence. In the context of person-centredness, competence is more than simply undertaking a task or demonstrating a desired behaviour,

Figure 4.1 Attributes of the nurse.

- professionally competent
- developed interpersonal skills
- commitment to the job
- clarity of beliefs and values
- knowing self

but is more reflective of a holistic approach that encompasses knowledge, skills and attitudes. The following definition of competence, provided by the Northern Ireland Practice and Education Council (2006) serves as a useful starting point:

> Competence is the combination of knowledge, skills, attitudes, values and judgement, which results in performance that satisfies a range of expected competencies (p. 8).

There are appropriate and relevant competencies for a nurse that are reflected in many competency frameworks reported in the literature, the most important being those produced by the regulatory bodies who govern the profession. The implicit assumption within the PCN Framework is that the minimum standards for registration will be met by any practicing nurse. For example, within the United Kingdom, the Nursing and Midwifery Council (NMC) set standards for the education of nurses, midwives and specialist community public health nurses and has identified core competencies that must be met during their training programme. Following registration, however, there is a requirement on nurses to continue to learn and develop, and to acquire skills that enable them to become more expert in practice. Benner's (1984) seminal work, based on the work of Dreyfus and Dreyfus (1986), describes five stages that nurses move through as they acquire mastery following registration: novice, advanced beginner, competent, proficient and expert. In summary, Dreyfus and Dreyfus (1986) explain the different levels as follows:

- As a *novice* the individual learns to rely on objective facts and from this determines rules that define action.
- At the stage of *advanced beginner* the individual has gained experience of coping with real situations and gaining more experience enables the processing of situations as a set of facts.
- The *competent* performer is able to determine the importance of some facts as dependent on the presence of other facts.
- The *proficient* performer makes decisions after reflecting on various options based on previous experience.
- The *expert* arrives at decisions based on 'mature and practiced understandings' (p. 30).

Benner's model has been used widely within nursing, with many examples available from the literature. For example, recent work conducted within Northern Ireland, referred to as the Clinical Careers Framework (CCF), has used Benner's model for skill acquisition within the context of lifelong learning and continuous professional development (McCormack et al., 2004; Boomer et al., 2006). The aim of the CCF is to offer a pathway for lifelong learning to enable practitioners to achieve their maximum potential. Within this initiative the five stages of skill acquisition are interpreted as follows:

1. *Novice* is the newly qualified nurse.
2. *Advanced beginner* is able to work within a team, mostly unsupervised, and manages a caseload of patients.

3. *Competent* practitioner is able to be a team leader and is aware of professional role and that of others.
4. *Proficient* practitioner who is able to manage the ward, staff and patients and affect the culture of the ward for practice development.
5. *Expert* practitioner is able to integrate global (i.e. corporate, national and international) input into issues relating to ward practice and creates a culture that fosters empowerment and effective evidence-based practice.

These stages were reflected in an Attributes Framework, with the focus being on developing practice expertise. The appraisal system was the vehicle used to self-assess and to gain feedback from others through a 360-degree feedback process in order to identify individual learning needs and learning opportunities.

Consistent with Benner's perspective, the authors of the CCF do not place emphasis on 'demonstrating competence in particular tasks or clinical procedures', but rather on the importance of technical expertise as 'embodied knowledge' (McCormack et al., 2004: 16). There does, however, tend to be an explicit focus on technical competence within the nursing literature, particularly from the perspective of the patient. The caring literature, for example, highlights a difference in perception between nurses and patients on what they consider to be the most important caring behaviours. A good example of this is the cohort of studies that have used the Caring Assessment Report Evaluation Q-Sort (CARE-Q) (Larson, 1981; Keane et al., 1987; Mayer, 1987; Komorita et al., 1991; Mangold, 1991; von Essen & Sjoden, 1991; Rosenthal, 1992). The CARE-Q indicated a notable difference between perceptions of patients and nurses, regarding what they considered as important nurse caring behaviours. Nurses tended to focus on the behaviours that would be indicative of the *care about* dimension such as listens to the patient (captured in the PCN Framework under developed interpersonal skills), whilst patients focused on those behaviours indicative of the *care for* dimension. Interestingly, the most important behaviour ranked by patient groups was *knows how to give shots, IVs, etc.* (captured in the PCN Framework under holistic care as providing for physical needs). Several qualitative studies exploring the meaning of caring also highlight the importance of technical competence from the perspective of patients, identifying themes related to provision of physical and/or technical competence (Brown, 1986; Ray, 1987; Vincent et al., 1996; McCance, 2003).

We can speculate on the reasons why patients focus on the technical aspects of care. Is it because patients feel safe in the hands of a nurse who is visibly competent in the 'tasks' she undertakes? Is it because the focus of care delivery is largely on routine and the completion of a series of often unrelated tasks? Is it because patients' first priority is their physical condition and symptom management and feeling physically better. Calman (2006), in a study using grounded theory, reports that patients describe competent nursing practice as a combination of technical care and nursing knowledge, but it is

The most common thing we hear when trying to implement change is that we 'don't have time for that'. The change to a culture of person-centred care has demonstrated how staff can make time for the small things that can make such an improvement to the quality of life of patients. Staff are taking time to facilitate life-stories, to listen to patients' choices and to engage in meaningful ways.

only when technical care is assumed that interpersonal attributes become the more important indicators of quality nursing care:

> Knowledge and technical skills are threshold competencies which are necessary for individuals to meet job requirements, but skill acquisition does not guarantee effective performance. Nurses need personal attributes and characteristics to translate hard facts, skills and knowledge into effective action.

(Calman, 2006: 721)

Alternatively, McCance et al. (1997) suggests Maslow's hierarchy of needs as a possible explanation for the differing perceptions held by nurses and patients. Maslow's theory proposes that it is only when the basic physical needs are met, such as effective pain relief, that patients can focus on other aspects of care. Irrespective of what a patient considers most important, it is incumbent on the nurse to get to know the patient and what is important to them during their care experience in order to deliver care that is person-centred. Nevertheless, the impact of nurses who are perceived to have poor technical skills can leave a vivid and lasting memory for patients and their families as illustrated by a participant in the study conducted by Vincent et al. (1996).

> *They're good nurses and they know their jobs. But yesterday a new nurse came in, and she actually asked me to take the blood sugar. She voiced the fact to us, the parents, that she didn't know what she was doing. She just said, "I don't know, it's been a long time since I took a blood sugar", and when she got to fumbling around, I said "Oh no", and did it myself, because I had watched the other nurses take it.*
>
> *(Vincent et al., 1996: 198, 199)*

From the perspective of the nurse, Conway (1996) would argue that expertise develops in response to the worldview held by practitioners and describes four worldviews that relate to how they use knowledge – technologists, traditionalists, specialists and humanistic existentialists. Technologists were considered to use a wide range of knowledge including anticipatory, diagnostic, technical (know how) and monitoring. Traditionalists were considered to be more concerned with survival, and therefore mainly referred to medical knowledge. Specialists were viewed as using knowledge of assessment, diagnosis and quality of life within a specific field of practice. They also had a transformative ability to extend their role as clinical nurse specialists. The humanistic existentialists were viewed as operating from a holistic practice perspective, which was concerned with values and drawing on theoretical knowledge and previous experience, underpinned by nursing and the social sciences. Conway refers to the impact of organisational culture and how this can act as a process of selection, promoting one perspective over another. Conway revealed that in some organisations where technical expertise was considered important, knowledge use and development was considered important to survive at a basic level, whilst in other organisations, where a worldview was more accepting of human development, expertise was considered on a more sophisticated level.

Irrespective of an individual's worldview, there is an expectation that nurses will continue to develop their competence throughout their career and become expert at what they do. There has, however, been much debate in the nursing literature on what constitutes expert nursing, (Benner, 1984; Manley et al., 2005, 2009), and whilst Benner's work has gone some way in describing the journey from novice to expert, we are still not entirely sure what nursing expertise looks like in practice (Baumann, 2006). The Royal College of Nursing's Expertise in Practice Project (Manley et al., 2005), building on the work of Manley and McCormack (1997), has made a significant contribution in this area through the identification of five attributes of expertise, which are described in Table 4.1.

Table 4.1 Attributes of expertise

Attribute	Description
Holistic practice knowledge	• using all forms of knowledge in practice • ongoing learning and evaluation from new situations • drawing from the range of knowledge bases (alongside experiential learning) to assess situations and inform appropriate action with consideration of consequences • embedding new knowledge and accessing this in similar situations as they occur
Saliency	• picking up cues that can be missed or dismissed by others to inform situations • observation of non-verbal cues to understand the person's individual situation • listening and responding to verbal cues; • regarding the patient as a whole (i.e. recognising their uniqueness) to inform treatment process • ability to recognise the needs of the patient, colleagues and others in the actions taken
Knowing the patient	• respect for people and their own view on the world (ontology) • respecting patient's unique perspective on their illness/situation • willingness to promote and maintain a person's dignity at all times • conscious use of self to promote a helping relationship • promoting the patient's own decision-making • willingness to relinquish 'control' to the patient • recognising the patient's/other's expertise
Moral agency	• providing information that will enhance people's ability to problem solve and make decisions for themselves • working at a level of consciousness that promotes another persons' dignity, respect and individuality • a conscientious awareness in one's work of integrity and impeccability • working and living one's values and beliefs, whilst not enforcing them on others
Skilled know-how	• enabling others through a willingness to share knowledge and skills • adapting and responding with consideration to each individual situation • mobilising and using all available resources • envisioning a path through a problem/situation and inviting others on that journey

(Manley et al., 2009: 6)

These attributes are person-centred in their orientation and are consistent with the philosophical principles underpinning the PCN Framework. For example, knowing the patient is a fundamental underpinning principle for the delivery of effective person-centred care and requires competence at a number of different levels that enables engagement with patients/clients and their families. Within the PCN Framework this is closely linked to person-centred processes, namely working with patients' beliefs and values and shared decision-making. The description of saliency is closely aligned to the acquisition of highly developed interpersonal skills, which for the purposes of the PCN Framework has been separated out from professional competence simply because it is a skill set that is considered fundamental to person-centred ways of working. Developed interpersonal skills are discussed in more detail in the following section. Similarly, moral agency reflects other attributes of the nurse identified in the Framework, the most notable being clarity of beliefs and values and knowing self. Working and living one's own values, whilst desirable, can be challenging to achieve in the real work of practice, particularly when the influence of the care environment is not conducive to a person-centred philosophy. (Refer to Chapter 5 for further discussion on the context of care.)

The following story provides an example of a nurse who displays a range of knowledge, skills, values and attitudes that characterise expert practice. This story illustrates elements within the care environment that can be a challenge to delivering optimal care, such as staff relationships and the issue of power. Expert practice, however, is also about being resourceful and implementing strategies required to manage the care environment in order to ensure effective person-centred care.

Mike is a 75-year-old man, admitted to the accident and emergency department having been found in a collapsed state on a side street of the local town. He had a long history of alcohol abuse and was known to the department for treatment of various minor injuries. Nurse Pigott received Mike into the department and took him to a cubicle for assessment. She knew Mike as a regular attender to the A&E department. Mike was a labourer who had travelled around the country working where he could. In 1984 Mike had fallen from some scaffolding and sustained serious injuries resulting in 8 months of hospitalisation. Following this his marriage broke up due to Mike's heavy drinking.

Nurse Pigott did some observations of Mike's vital signs and found: pulse 100 per min, blood pressure 160/90 and temperature 36.5°C (ax). His pupils were equal and reacting to light. There were scars on his left arm and leg. Mike was very talkative as usual, although his voice was very slurred. Nurse Pigott 'felt' that his speech sounded different this time, although she knew he had been drinking heavily.

Mike was examined by the department's doctor, who also attempted to perform a neurological examination. Due to Mike's inebriated state he was unable to co-operate fully with this examination. However, the doctor felt sure that Mike's fall was due to his alcohol consumption and therefore felt that Mike could be discharged 'when he had slept it off'.

Nurse Pigott was not convinced about the doctor's diagnosis and discussed her anxieties about Mike's speech with him. The doctor could not see grounds for nurse Pigott's concerns and insisted Mike be discharged as soon as possible. Nurse Pigott took her case to the senior nurse, who intervened on her behalf and eventually persuaded the doctor to allow Mike to stay in the assessment ward overnight, to be re-assessed the following morning.

Next morning Mike tried to get out of bed to visit the toilet and fell to the floor. He was unable to support himself on his left leg and he was 'carrying' his left arm. The physicians were called to see Mike, and on examination diagnosed him with a left-sided cerebrovascular accident.

(McCormack, 1992: 342, 343)

Developed Interpersonal Skills

The nature of person-centredness as that which focuses on relationships indicates the need for a strong interpersonal skill base. McCormack and McCance (2006) describe developed interpersonal skills as 'the ability of the nurse to communicate at a variety of levels' (p. 475). Effective communication requires a combination of good verbal and non-verbal skills. Verbal communication deals with what is said (speech), and what is heard (listening) whilst non-verbal communication is concerned with body language such as posture, proximity and touch and movements, facial expressions, eye contact gestures and other behaviours, which can add another layer of communication to verbal messages. There are many nursing texts available that focus on these fundamental communication skills, however, we would argue that person-centred communication is more than the sum of its parts and that each interaction is dependent on the people involved. In essence we communicate with individuals based on what we know about them as people. This will influence what we say, how we say it, the language used and the use of strategies. Getting this right is really important because the impact of poor interpersonal communication can be profound and often increases the vulnerability experienced by patients, which is clearly demonstrated in the study by Reiman (1986).

Developing person-centred ways of working has been like becoming familiar with using a mobile phone! I am not very technical minded and therefore initially I would only use my phone when I had to or when required – a little like person-centred practice. But as I became more familiar with it, I felt it was part of me. I could not go anywhere without it, it became part of me, part of who I am – like person-centred practice, a great way to engage, a tool I can not do without, I think of it all the time.

> *She was always in a hurry, she didn't have time to talk or even if she had time she didn't really seem to want to talk. Her body language let me know she wasn't interested in what I had to say. All she was here to do was to perform her duty and go home. She stood at a distance, she didn't even come close. She made me feel I have some kind of illness and I might rub off on her. When I was talking to her she wouldn't look at me directly. When I would ask her a question she would be snappy even on the defensive side. She wasn't interested in the person as a whole. She would cut me off short and she talked in such a rush. She never would say when she'd be back. I was not at ease. I was uncomfortable. I became depressed by not being able to talk. I felt I had to keep my mouth shut.*
>
> *(Reiman, 1986)*

The development of effective interpersonal ability is linked to the notion of emotional intelligence. Historically, intelligence has been based on the assessment of a person's 'intelligence quotient' (IQ). To a large extent, this is still the case and education systems continue to use this as the yardstick of cognitive ability and intellect. Goleman (1999) argues that education systems worldwide are geared to valuing and developing these capacities at the expense of other capabilities, such as the ability to get on with other people. Howard Gardner challenged these assumptions in his book *Frames of Mind*. Gardner (1993) argued that 'my intelligence does not stop at my skin' and suggested that we have a 'spectrum of intelligences' as well as the logical–mathematical and linguistic capabilities traditionally thought of as intelligence. Gardner suggested that:

> *Inter*personal intelligence is the ability to understand other people: what motivates them, how they work, how to work cooperatively with them. Successful salespeople, politicians, teachers, clinicians, and religious leaders are all likely to be individuals with high degrees of interpersonal intelligence. *Intra*personal intelligence . . . is a correlative ability, turned inward. It is a capacity to form an accurate, veridical model of oneself and to be able to use that model to operate effectively in life.

(Gardner, 1993: 9; cited in Goleman, 1996: 39)

What this quote of emotional intelligence highlights is that using emotions intelligently is a combination of knowing 'self' and knowing 'others' in the context of emotional beings, that is how I and others that I relate to respond emotionally. It is through an understanding of 'self' as an emotional being that we can respond effectively to the emotional behaviours of others. This is also an important element within the PCN Framework articulated as 'clarity of beliefs and values' and 'knowing self'.

Weisinger (1998) suggests that emotional intelligence is derived from four basic elements that operate like the building blocks of DNA. If nurtured with experience, these elements can enable the development of specific skills and abilities in using emotions intelligently. Psychologists John Mayer and Peter Salovey developed the concept of 'emotional intelligence' as being made up of these four building blocks. These building blocks represent abilities or skills. They are hierarchical, with each level incorporating and building upon the capabilities of all previous ones (Weisinger, 1998). The four building blocks are:

1. The ability to accurately perceive, appraise and express emotion.
2. The ability to access or generate feelings on demand when they can facilitate understanding of yourself or another person.
3. The ability to understand emotions and the knowledge that derives from them.
4. The ability to regulate emotions to promote emotional and intellectual growth.

Peter Salovey developed these into five competencies or skills and these have been popularised through the work of Daniel Goleman (1996, 1999), which are described as follows:

1. *self-awareness* – knowing one's internal states, preferences resources and intuitions
2. *self-regulation* – managing one's internal states, impulses and resources
3. *motivation* – emotional tendencies that guide or facilitate reaching goals
4. *empathy* – awareness of others' feelings, emotions or concerns
5. *social skills* – adeptness at inducing desirable responses in others
(Goleman, 1999: 26, 27).

The following example is drawn from the Expertise in Practice Project (Manley et al., 2005), and describes a nurse who demonstrates competencies aligned to emotional intelligence. This example also demonstrates the impact of this practitioner on the care environment, his patients and working colleagues.

> He is caring for staff as well, he knows the rules and regulations, he's very professional He has empathy and that also transfers into his staff. He is like a role model in a way. He is well respected, I think the consultants respect him very much as well, the way he deals with everybody . . . he is very helpful, giving help and direction with it. Apart from all that staff go to him for personal and professional advice. He's confidential, he's a good all rounder. He supports the medical staff, he won't be critical, but if people are not performing properly he'll take over in a way that makes you feel relaxed . . . He welcomes everybody into the department, we call him 'the welcomer'! If a patient is hostile, he 's very calming. He doesn't shout, he's got a way with people. He could stop a volatile situation developing.
>
> (Manely et al., 2005: 18)

Goleman (1999) views emotional intelligence as central to leadership and defines a leader as an individual who can get others to do their job more effectively. He states that ineptitude in leaders 'wastes time, creates acrimony, corrodes motivation and commitment, builds hostility and apathy' (p. 32). This is particularly pertinent in the context of nursing, with a growing evidence base focusing on leadership styles, the qualities of transformational leaders and their impact on culture, which is discussed in detail in Chapter 5. Furthermore, the competence of nurses particularly in relation to interpersonal communication has been drawn out in a recent qualitative study by McCabe (2004), who concluded that nurses can communicate well with patients when they use a person-centred approach, but the ability to do so is heavily influenced by the work and culture of the organisation, that is the care environment. This supports the relationship between the skills of the nurse as a pre-requisite for managing the care environment in order to deliver person-centred care, as depicted in the PCN Framework.

Points to Ponder

Identify one person in your team who you consider is a good role model. What attributes do they demonstrate and how do these relate to the PCN Framework?

Being Committed to the Job

Being committed to the job at the most basic level reflects 'dedication and a sense that the nurse wants to provide care that is best for the patient' (McCormack & McCance, 2006: 475). The idea of personal commitment at an individual level is reflected in a number of qualitative studies exploring caring in nursing. Various theme labels were identified across these studies such as: *beyond the call of duty (Ford, 1990); giving of self (Chipman, 1991); level of motivation* (Morrison, 1991); *going the extra mile* (Fosbinder, 1994) and *the extra touch* (McCance, 2003). All these themes describe nurses who act not because they are expected to, but because they want to. McCance (1999) and Binnie and Titchen (1999) provide the following descriptions of nurses who are perceived as being committed to their job.

> *. . . I don't know like, but most of them I got on great with, but there was just something about her that I couldn't, she just, it was as if she was just there because I suppose she needed a job, where the rest of them seemed to put their heart and soul into it you know. They seemed to be more sort of dedicated and would have sat and you know if you had said something was worrying you, they would have sat and talked to you . . . .*
>
> *(McCance, 1999: 183)*

> *Many nurses came in early or stayed late to do something particular with a patient or to finish important work for which they felt personally responsible. . . . Far from abusing the freedom they were given to manage their time, the nurses tended to give more time to the ward than they had done previously and than was 'officially' required.*
> *(Binnie Titchen, 1999: 108)*

Commitment to the job can also be linked to the idea of intentionality, a term that is often used interchangeably with other terms such as intention, intent or will (Malinski, 2009). The concept of intentionality is discussed in the caring literature by several nurse theorists. Watson (1985) defines caring as 'a value and an attitude that has to become a will, an intention or a commitment that manifests itself in concrete acts' (p. 32). Furthermore, she believes that 'our intentionalities inform our choices and actions, helping us to be sensitive and mindful about what is most important in our lives and work' (p. 17). Similarly, Boykin and Schoenhoffer (1993) define caring as 'the intentional and authentic presence of the nurse with another who is recognised as person living caring and growing in caring' (p. 25). Malinski (2009) in her philosophical commentary on intentionality and consciousness highlights the risk of bringing about a particular outcome as a goal of the practitioner, as opposed to gaols that are determined by the person. This is an important idea in the context of person-centred care and is well illustrated by Schoenhoffer (2002) who uses the following story to explore the meaning of intentionality and how it relates to personhood.

I pulled up to the singlewide trailer in the migrant camp with the intent of speaking to a parent regarding her child's excessive absences. What I saw when I pulled up was school age children everywhere. I noticed one child in particular. She looked to be about 5 or 6 years of age. She wasn't quite as pretty as the other children. She was very dirty and had long hair that hung in her eyes. She was holding a very dirty puppy that had no hair. It looked almost dead. She was hugging and kissing the puppy and telling it that she loved it.

As I got out of the car, all of the children ran to the trailer door to tell their parents that someone was there, all except for the one little girl. She walked up to me and asked me if I liked her puppy. She had so much love in her eyes for this dog.

A woman came to the door and one of her older children translated for us. At first, I sensed that she was very uneasy talking to me and did not want to say very much. I felt desperate and really wanted to help this family. It appeared as if about 20 people were living here. In the meantime, the little girl handed me her puppy and I took it. The little girl hugged me and said, "take it home and make it fat and all better". I could not say no to her (I did

(Continued)

take the puppy home and it did get better). The little girl was so sincere. Something happened that changed everything. This mother's whole attitude changed.

She opened up to me and revealed many things about her family's situation that enabled me to help them. I fell in love with this entire family. All of the kids are now in school and they are living in their own trailer. Local resources helped feed them through the winter months because crops had been frozen out.

I see this little girl often, and every time I see her she runs up to me and hugs me and gives me the softest, sweetest kiss on the cheek and tells me that she loves me. She also tells me that I am her best friend.

(Schoenhoffer, 2002: 37)

This nurse went into this situation with a very specific goal but her interaction with the child and the family took her on different journey. Schoenhoffer (2002) infers that 'the intentionality of the nurse consisted of more than simple intent, but involved commitment an openness to larger possibilities' (p. 36). Reflected in this account is a commitment from the nurse to do what is right for the family, which did not align with the goal that she started out with. Intentionality, and the commitment that this reveals, is also linked to personal values. Schoenhoffer (2002) comments: 'commitment involves more than mere intent – it implies devotion and action – sending oneself out into the world in active expression of one's avowed values' (p. 39).

For person-centredness to be effective a variety of committed individuals are required, all with a different energy to bring to it. When these people are energised and they mix their individual energies together the result is beautiful.

Commitment to the job can also be demonstrated within teams, and indeed it is within a team structure that we deliver care. Demonstrating commitment at team level can be challenging, particularly if the team is not functioning effectively. Research from Aston University by Borrill et al. (1999) suggests that the quality of teamworking is powerfully related to:

- clear team objectives
- high level of participation within the team
- high level of commitment to quality
- high levels of support for innovation

Furthermore, Borrill et al. (1999) report a significant and negative relationship between the percentage of staff working in teams and mortality rates with the hospital studied. In other words where more employees work in teams the mortality rates appear to be lower.

The contemporary leadership literature also emphasises the importance of transformational leadership, where leaders focus on people and problem-solving in an environment of constant change (Bass, 1985). Transformational leaders as described by Kouzes and Posner (2002a) 'enable others to act', by embracing approaches that foster collaboration, building trust and providing visible support. Such approaches enable leaders to integrate their roles of clinical expert, practice developer, resource manager and leader (Manley, 2000b). It is also accepted that in healthcare there is a correlation between the quality of patient care, staff morale and effective nursing leadership (Cunningham and Kitson, 2000c). The Commission for Health Improvement's (CHI) review of service failures identified inadequate clinical leadership and poor team relationships as the most common risk factors at operational level (www.chi.gov.uk).

Within practice development a fundamental activity for team effectiveness is ensuring clarity of beliefs and values, which is central to developing a shared vision. It is this that can then provide a clear purpose that everyone can sign up to. According to the RCN (2007): 'a vision is shared when two or more practitioners have a similar image or mental picture of what they want to create and are committed to one another and to making it happen' (p. 4.1). Developing a shared vision, as the corner stone to enable teams to deliver effective person-centred care practice, is demonstrated through the projects presented in Chapter 8. A cohesive team with a shared purpose can be very powerful as illustrated by the following example.

> John was a 76-year-old man who had been admitted to hospital for symptom management following a recent diagnosis of lung cancer. He had no close relatives and after a few days of being in hospital the nursing staff soon realised that John received very few visitors apart from his local priest. Ann, a senior nurse within the team, was caring for John one morning and was talking to him about his life, only to discover that he had been a prisoner in a concentration camp during the Second World war. John talked about his experience openly and what he had endured during that time. Ann was struck by the dignity John displayed in the face of extreme adversity and shared John's life story with the other members of the nursing team. This enabled everyone to gain an understanding of John and what was important to him in his life. John, however, deteriorated very quickly and was soon requiring end of life care. The nursing team were aware that John received few visitors and everyone shared the same goal – they didn't want John to die alone. The team set about putting in place a rota that allowed a nurse to sit with John at all times, except when the priest visited, which was often. The consequences of this decision meant that there was one less member of staff available to work with the remainder of the patients on the ward, but because this was a shared decision by the team no one complained. John did not die alone and passed away peacefully in the company of his priest.

Commitment to the job should also be considered in the context of organisational commitment and their relationship to job satisfaction. Blegen (1993) describes job satisfaction in terms of the degree of positive orientation the individual has towards their job. In Blegen's (1993) meta-analysis of job satisfaction, 48 studies were analysed with a combined sample size of 15,048 subjects. From the findings Blegen identified 13 variables that were consistently reported in all quantitative studies. Four of these were personal attributes such as age, education and years of experience and the remaining nine combined organisation traits and sources of stress. Blegen reported that job satisfaction was most closely associated with stress and organisational commitment. Furthermore, it is suggested from the literature that organisational commitment is influenced by organisational culture, and understanding organisational culture is important because it influences how we view organisational life and organisational activities (Manley, 2001). Workplace culture has a big influence on the care environment and the key point to make is that strong cultures are often associated with superior organisational performance. This is dealt with in detail within Chapter 5. Smith and Clutterbuck (1984) suggest that the strength of a culture is the product of two factors:

1. sharedness, which is the extent of shared core values throughout the organisation
2. intensity, which is the degree of commitment of all employees in the organisation to these values.

This emphasises the relationship between commitment to the job and clarity of beliefs and values not just at individual level, but at team and organisational levels.

Clarity of Beliefs and Values

The PCN Framework identifies clarity of beliefs and values as one of the pre-requisites that enables practitioners to work with the care environment. According to Manley (2004), 'values determine what people think *ought* to be done (p. 55)' and these are closely linked with moral and ethical codes. For example, a value could be: *people have a right to be treated as individuals with their own life history.* Beliefs on the other hand are 'what people think is true or not true' (p. 55). For example, a belief could be: *taking account of patients' preferences increases their satisfaction with care.* Beliefs and values are interrelated in that 'it is difficult to separate values from their believed effect' (p. 55). In the earlier example *taking account of patients' preferences* is the value, but the belief is that this *increases their satisfaction with care.* Finally, basic assumptions involve beliefs, interpretation of beliefs plus values and emotions and are understood as accepted truths that are held unconsciously and are taken for granted (Brown, 1998). For example, *practitioners working in a team might assume that all patients in their ward are treated with respect and their preferences are taken into consideration.* One cannot question the values and beliefs underpinning this assumption, but one should be able to observe them in action, that is, how they are played out in the behaviours of the team members. The challenge arises when espoused values (i.e. the values we talk about) do not match the behaviours we see in practice.

The story presented below is an extract from the work of Binnie and Titchen (1999), which focused on the introduction of primary nursing in one medical ward over a 3-year-period. This story is a reflective account from a staff nurse who was involved in this project and demonstrates the values and beliefs held by this nurse. One of her implicit value was that *nurses spending time caring for patients is good nursing practice*. She believed that *a patient-centred approach to care would achieve this*, and she assumed that *this was the everyday practice taking place on her ward*. Her story, however, tells something different – the values she espoused and the reality of practice where incongruent. Nonetheless, her story reflects a significant journey towards 'enlightenment', which according to Fay (1987), involves becoming aware of taken for granted aspects of everyday life and becoming aware of them through consciousness-raising. Her realisation of how she had been practicing had risen to a conscious level, and she was then able to change her approach to managing her workload.

When I think about PCN I think about a 'recordable DVD'. In life we love to be able to record memorable events so that we can have them to look back on, to be able to keep them close to our hearts – the same way that I hope PCN can be kept within our hearts (like a DVD) and that we can keep it forever.

Camouflaged Task-Oriented Nursing

On Saturday . . . I was on a late . . . At about 5 p.m. I suddenly realized that I was working the shift in a way I'd not done before. Instead of rushing around doing all the outstanding things which I needed doing, such as taking out a ventflon, organising transport, etc., I was actually going around my patients giving them all the nursing care I could.

I suppose I'd moved on from organising my work around tasks that needed doing and was actually organising my time around the patients and therefore doing those tasks which I had to do, but also nursing the person at the same time – incorporating the tasks into my care. And so I . . . walked Elizabeth down the ward and back instead of just giving her tablets, etc.

I don't know why I suddenly started working in this way – perhaps because I've found the confidence to stop rushing around trying to do the things I have to do and found that I could slow down and give the care I should be giving . . . Despite being saturated with the patient-centred approach to nursing care and . . . finding task-oriented nursing an anathema, I hadn't realized that I was actually working in a task-oriented style! I'm incredibly surprised, not to say somewhat horrified, that I have been working from such a bad basis of practice! In theory, I totally rejected task-centred care and yet I suddenly realise that my practice has been task-centred, although so well camouflaged that I hadn't even realized. [Barbara]

(Binnie & Titchen, 1999: 108)

The idea of clarifying personal beliefs and values is a way of articulating and making explicit what we believe ought to be done and what we understand to be true. Within practice development this is often achieved through the use of a Values Clarification Exercise (VCE), a tool used to produce an explicit statement of values and belief (Warfield & Manley, 1990). This vision statement or ward philosophy can then be used to challenge practice in an environment that is supportive and is committed to learning in and from practice. Wright and McCormack (2001) comment that the ward philosophy should act as a 'standard to aim for during the change process' (p. 39). VCE uses processes that are collaborative and require engagement thus increasing a sense of ownership.

The link between clarifying values and believes and workplace culture is clearly described by Manley (2004):

> Values and beliefs contribute to shared meanings, understandings and expectations which are tacit and distinctive to a particular group and passed on to new members. . . . they underpin the way things are done within any cultural focus (p. 54).

This can further explain why Barbara in the previous story found herself in a position of practising in a task-oriented way. The ward had become focused on the busyness and the tasks that were expected to be completed by the end of each shift, and that had become the cultural norm. This reinforces the importance of reflecting in and on practice, which if undertaken within a mentorship relationship has the potential to uncover strongly held personal and professional values and beliefs and enhance understanding of our own actions and the influence of culture. The impact of workplace culture on person-centred care is discussed in greater detail in Chapter 5. Furthermore, the use of practice development as an approach that can facilitate clarity of values and beliefs in order to be able to work with the culture and context, to deliver effective person-centred care is discussed in greater detail in the final chapter.

Points to Ponder

What values and beliefs do you hold about nursing and how do they influence your practice? What values and belief do others in your team hold about nursing and how do you know?

Knowing Self

The idea of clarifying personal beliefs and values is closely connected to knowing self, and as indicated by McCormack and McCance (2006) is based on the assumption that 'before we can help others we need to have insight into how we function as a person' (p. 475). In Chapter 2 we explored the concept of person, which we have argued captures the attributes that represent our humanness, that is, how we think about moral values, and how we express political, spiritual or religious beliefs. These attributes then shape how we develop relationships and how we engage at an emotional level. Furthermore, we grow as persons during our lifetime through engagement with the social world, and it is this that informs our personal meanings, beliefs and values and determines 'who I am'. In the context of the PCN Framework, this infers that the way an individual sees him/herself, and the way they construct their world can influence how they practice as a nurse and how they engage with patients.

In a review of the literature on the value of nursing, Horton et al. (2007) identify a body of research that suggests personal value systems influence professional lifestyle, and applying this to nursing state 'nurses' personal value systems influence the actions they take' (p. 724). Horton et al. (2007) conclude that the evidence reinforces the need for nurses to have a clear understanding of their own values. McCormack (2003) in his original framework refers to 'nurses' value history' and relates this to decision-making, suggesting that a nurses' own value system can influence the decisions made by patients at an unconscious or indeed conscious level. McCormack (2003) argues:

> If a mutual relationship exists between the nurse and the patient, then it is especially important that the nurse's values are expressed, particularly when they conflict with the patient's values (p. 206).

The value of knowing self is illustrated through the work undertaken by Masterson (2007) with community matrons. This is a role developed within the United Kingdom that focuses on caseload management with patients who are chronically ill (DoH, 2005). She places her discussion in the context of courageous conversations that for community matrons often involve disagreement, disappointment and/or bad news. Positive outcomes are therefore reliant on 'both participants being prepared to learn and having a genuine curiosity about the other person's perspective' (p. 30). Masterson discusses the idea of having conversations that can trigger an emotional response resulting from our own life history. This can subsequently result in undesired actions that can impact on the process of engaging with patients (refer to Chapter 6). The following story is an example of the impact personal life experiences can have on our practice and the importance of being open to our limitations.

One useful model for exploring and understanding self in the context of relationships is The *Johari Window* (Luft, 1984), which is

Patricia was a nurse who had worked in palliative care for 10 years. She was committed to her work and recognised the privileged position she held when working with patients who were dying and their families. She was recognised by her colleagues as an expert practitioner who had the ability to get to know her patients, recognising their needs and knowing what was important to them at the most distressing time in their lives. That was until Patricia's own mother was diagnosed with ovarian cancer, detected at a very late stage.

(Continued)

Patricia took a leave of absence to look after her mother who deteriorated very rapidly and eventually died 2 months later. Patricia had always been very close to her mum and her death was almost unbearable, but she returned to work soon after her bereavement in an attempt to 'get back to normal'. She assumed her own loss would further enhance her understanding of the pain and suffering experienced by her patients and their families. Patricia, however, was not prepared for the impact her work was to have on her personal well-being. Every patient she met, every interaction she had with grieving families was a painful reminder of her own loss. Patricia recognised she was not coping and discussed her issues with her clinical supervisor. She realised that because of her own life experience she did not have the emotional reserves to provide the best care to her patients. This was inconsistent with Patricia's value and beliefs about high quality nursing care, which eventually led to her decision to request a transfer to another clinical area.

presented in Figure 4.2. Interaction between two or more people depends on the degree to which people can be open and the context in which it takes place. The window describes the possible forms of awareness, behaviour and feelings in a relationship using four quadrants.

Quadrant 1: This refers to the behaviours, feelings and motivations that I know about myself and others are aware of too. These behaviours are open to all to see and we willingly display them.

Quadrant 2: This refers to the behaviours, feelings and motivations that others see but I don't. I display behaviours that others can see but I am not aware of them. I believe I am displaying my public self (Quadrant 1) but the person/people I am interacting with can see my public self but also can see elements of my 'blind self'. An example may be to do with values, where I verbalise a particular belief, but my actual behaviour is inconsistent with the belief expressed.

Quadrant 3: This is the hidden area and represents feelings, behaviours and motivations that I am aware of but am unwilling to convey to others.

Quadrant 4: This is the segment that I do not know about and others do not know either. Dreams and visions often give us insight into some of these areas.

It is argued that our interactions can become more effective when we become aware of our feelings, motivations and behaviours and when we move more to Quadrant 1. Facilitated self-reflection is an important mechanism for increasing our self-awareness and understanding our behaviours. The importance of reflecting on what you are doing, as part of the learning process, has been emphasised by many investigators. Schon (1983) suggests that the capacity to

	Known to self	Not known to self
Known to others	1 **Open**	2 **Blind**
Not known to others	3 **Hidden**	4 **Unknown**

Figure 4.2 The Johari Window.

reflect on action so as to engage in a process of continuous learning is one of the defining characteristics of professional practice. Being able to reflect in action (whilst doing something) and on action (after you have done it) has become an important feature of professional training programmes in many disciplines. Mezirow (1991) refers to critical reflection and argues that it is important to reflect on assumptions and presuppositions (particularly about oneself) and that this in turn leads to what he calls 'transformative learning':

> Perspective transformation is the process of becoming critically aware of how and why our presuppositions have come to constrain the way we perceive, understand, and feel about our world; of reformulating these assumptions to permit a more inclusive, discriminating, permeable and integrative perspective; and of making decisions or otherwise acting on these new understandings. More inclusive, discriminating, permeable and integrative perspectives are superior perspectives that adults choose if they can because they are motivated to better understand the meaning of their experience (p. 14).

The importance of the role of mentor or professional supervisor within a reflective model is significant as is the case with clinical supervision, which is attracting significant interest within a variety of professional groupings (e.g. nursing, midwifery and social work). We would suggest that this interest is in recognition of the need for an approach that assists practitioners to develop their internal motivations for developing and providing quality approaches to their practice. Johns (1998) suggests that clinical supervision has a primary focus on achieving 'therapeutic electiveness' and that the role of the clinical supervisor is to facilitate a practitioner to do this by reflecting on their work experiences.

Supervision can be used to facilitate growth and development at different levels of the organisation. Essentially, the supervisor is somebody who 'facilitates growth' and provides essential support necessary for the practice of clinical excellence. The personal nature of supervision, as an individually focused activity, centring on the development needs of the individual, contributes to 'knowing self' in the context of being a practitioner.

Points to Ponder

What is your experience of clinical supervision and how could this approach be used to increase your practice expertise in providing person-centred care?

Summary of Key Points

The pre-requisites, as presented in the PCN Framework and discussed in this chapter, form the fundamental building blocks for achieving practice that is person-centred. As this chapter demonstrates the pre-requisites are not mutually exclusive but are interwoven, with close connections between all five elements. Competencies relate not only to technical ability, but also to emotional intelligence and leadership qualities that enable individuals to work in complex healthcare environments. Developed interpersonal skills are pivotal to the development of therapeutic relationships and we have attempted in this chapter to draw out elements of this skill base that play an important role in being person-centred as a way of being. Clarifying values and beliefs and knowing self are at the heart of person-centred care and places a responsibility on the nurse not just to get to know his/her patient, but to also recognise what they bring of themselves into the caring interaction. The Framework makes explicit the need for nurses to move beyond a focus on technical competence and requires nurses to engage in authentic humanistic caring practices that focus on personhood.

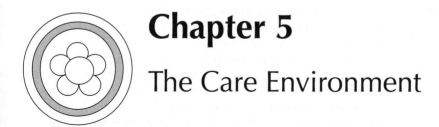

Chapter 5

The Care Environment

Introduction

In the previous chapter the attributes of the nurse, as pre-requisites for working in a person-centred way were discussed. However, irrespective of the characteristics of the nurse, unless the care environment is conducive to person-centred ways of working then these characteristics and potentials can't be fully realised. The care environment focuses on the context in which care is delivered. Increasingly, context is recognised as having a significant impact on clinical and team effectiveness. There is an increasing literature in the field of knowledge translation and knowledge utilisation exploring the meaning of context and the contextual factors that help or hinder the use of knowledge in practice. Many studies have attempted to delineate the key elements of context, explore particular elements of context and their enabling or hindering qualities (for evidence/knowledge use) and develop approaches to measuring the impact of context on clinical and team effectiveness, including impact on patient outcome. What the majority of studies recognise is that context is a complex phenomenon and whilst it may be easy to state what it is (in our case context refers to the care environment) less easy to delineate its characteristics and qualities. To some extent this difficulty relates to a debate about the relationship between context and culture and for some writers, it is more important to understand and evaluate culture and the way in which it is manifested in practice.

In this chapter we take the approach that context is synonymous with the 'care environment' and that contained within the environment of care are multifaceted characteristics and qualities of the environment (people, processes and structures) that impact on the effectiveness of PCN. Indeed in the articulation of the PCN Framework (Chapter 3) we have argued that the care environment has a significant

Figure 5.1 Characteristics of the care environment.

- skill mix
- shared decision-making systems
- staff relationships
- organisational systems
- power
- the potential for innovation and risk-taking
- the physical environment

impact on the operationalisation of PCN and has the greatest potential to limit or enhance the facilitation of person-centred processes. To this end, when we developed the PCN Framework, we identified six characteristics of the care environment that enhance or limit PCN. However, since the original development of the Framework, significant work has been undertaken to evaluate the impact of the care environment itself, that is the physical environment and so we have added this as an additional characteristic of the care environment construct (Figure 5.1).

These seven characteristics will be used to shape the structure of the chapter. However, before discussing these, the issue of workplace culture will be discussed in order to make the case that culture is not a 'thing' that a context has, but something that a context 'is' and that the culture is created and recreated by the actors in the context.

Workplace Culture

When we think about care practices it is hard to set these outside of a 'setting'. Irrespective of where we work as nurses, we are inevitably undertaking that practice in a setting – be it a hospital ward, a clinic, a community, a home. Each of these are care settings, that is places where people receive care and as such have cultural characteristics that help or hinder effectiveness in the receipt and delivery of care services. The literature on culture in health and social care is complex, broad and diverse. Manley (2004) has argued that some of the problems associated with understanding culture arise from a lack of distinction in the literature (and among decision-makers) between 'organisational culture' and 'workplace culture'.

Organisational culture in health and social care has been studied extensively over the past 20 years. This is not to suggest that culture was not of interest in the preceding years, but the international drive (particularly over the past 15 years) to 'modernise' health care systems has led to a significant focus on the impact of culture on the clinical effectiveness of staff and service-users experiences of health and social care. Examples of such modernisation programmes internationally include, 'the 1000 Lives Campaign Wales' (a national patient safety and clinical effectiveness campaign http://www.npsa.nhs.uk/nrls/improvingpatientsafety/campaigns/1000-lives-campaign-wales/); the National Health Service Institute for Innovation and Improvement (with a remit for supporting the NHS in England and Wales to transform health care for patients and the public by rapidly developing and spreading new ways of working, new technology and leadership http://www.institute.nhs.uk/); the Australian Council on Healthcare Standards (with a remit for quality standards and accreditation http://www.achs.org.au/); the Institute for Health Improvement (IHI) in the USA http://www.ihi.org (the IHI has a worldwide remit for improving health care

systems). What is consistent across all these modernisation programmes is the emphasis on changing the cultures of organisations,
of teams and of individual practices.

Davies et al. (2000) argue that whilst there are many conceptions
of culture, broadly, perspectives are divided between those that view
culture as something an organisation 'is' and those that view it as
something that an organisation 'has'. The former being characteristics of an organisation that are 'fixed', immutable and serve as
descriptors of an organisation. When an organisation is considered
to 'have' culture then these are 'aspects or variables of the organisation that can be isolated, described and manipulated' (p. 112). Davies
et al. (2000) argue that it is only through the view that organisations
'have culture' that it is possible to consider ways in which culture can
be changed. Schein (2004) suggests that in any organisation, there
are three levels in which the culture is manifested and experienced –
artefacts, espoused values and assumptions:

> *Artefacts (What is seen, heard and felt):* visible products, such as
> language, technology, clothing/uniforms, stories, myths, symbols,
> forms of address.
> *Espoused Values (What is lived):* the way in which individual
> and shared values are experienced (or not) in a team/care setting.
> *Basic Assumptions (What does it mean):* meanings of the cul-
> ture that emerge through the articulation of shared values and the
> validation, examination and meaning making through learning and
> repeated problem-solving.

Davies and others have argued that reforms in health care have
moved from focusing on the artefacts of organisations (such as
reorganising management layers) to dealing with the complex web
of basic assumptions that underpin the functioning of any health
care organisation (such as the amount of autonomy experienced by
professionals or the centrality of patients' values). However, if we
believe that organisations are merely manifestations of a carefully
(or not) woven web of cultural characteristics that can be manipulated, then we miss the complexity of culture as articulated by
Schein (2004) and we can treat people in the culture as 'pawns' that
can be manipulated to suit our/others ends. Instead, Manley (2004)
(after Bate, 1994) argues that organisations *are* cultures, incorporating such things as language, myths, rules and stories. Thomas
et al. (1990: 18) suggest that these aspects of culture are 'ways of
thinking, behaving and believing that members have in common'.
This more anthropological notion of culture likened to what Davies
et al. (2000) refer to as 'post-modern' understandings of culture,
whereby culture is not comprised of malleable elements, but instead
is something that is 'lived' by its members. However, all of us have
experience of being in a culture that has a particular set of espoused
beliefs, values and assumptions, but our experiences differ from
what is espoused. This is often a common experience for patients.

Evelyn, a 78-year-old woman was admitted via the emergency department for treatment following a fall resulting in a fractured hip. Whilst the organisation philosophy espoused a culture whereby patients' preferences would be considered alongside organisational commitments, Evelyn was very dissatisfied with her experience in hospital. She moved to three different wards during her hospital stay, she found it difficult to keep track of what her plan of treatment and care was as she had different care workers in and between care settings, she didn't feel that any one person *really* knew her home circumstances and staff continually failed to remember her daily routines and preferences. Whilst Evelyn was treated successfully and was helped to regain her mobility that allowed her to return to a semi-independent level of functioning, overall, Evelyn felt very dissatisfied with her hospital experience.

(Story based on interview data from McCormack et al., 2008)

The monitoring of patients' experiences of hospital services is now common place, but Manley (2000a) argues that accreditation systems have largely focused on how an organisation as a whole functions rather than getting inside the cultures of individual workplaces. She goes on to argue that the effectiveness of the organisation at large is dependent on the effectiveness of the individual settings (contexts) in which patients receive care and staff practice. Manley suggests that this (organisational culture) is not the culture that patients and staff experience everyday, instead, what they do experience is the culture of different settings (contexts) or workplaces. Wilson et al. (2005), Coeling and Simms (1993) and Adams and Bond (1997) have argued that there is a need to understand the culture of the individual workplace prior to implementing innovations or developments, as culture has been found to vary between units within the same organisation. Manley et al. argue that accreditation systems make the assumption that an organisational culture is an aggregate of individual unit/department (micro) cultures (often referred to as sub-cultures) whilst in reality these individual unit/department cultures can vary significantly. Thus, Manley (2004) adopts the term 'idio-culture' (after Bolan & Bolan, 1994) to argue the point that there are different cultures that exert an influence on each other rather than one organisational/corporate culture with sub-cultures within a hierarchical arrangement. One such idio-culture is a practice setting (workplace). McCormack, Manley and Walsh (2008: 22) define workplace culture as:

> the most immediate culture experienced and/or perceived by staff, patients, users and other key stakeholders. This is the culture that impacts directly on the delivery of care. It both influences and is influenced by the organisational and corporate cultures with which it interfaces as well as other idio-cultures through staff relationships and movement.

An effective workplace culture is one in which there is:

- A person-centred approach with patients, users and staff.
- Daily decision-making is transparent and evidence-based, where evidence is the blending of different sources of knowledge (patient preferences, empirical research, critical reflection of experience and professional expertise and local knowledge [e.g. audit findings]).
- A learning culture in which through formal critique there is a focus on individual, team and service effectiveness.
- Development of leadership potential to achieve a culture of empowerment, continuing modernisation and innovation.

(Manley, 2004: 2)

> David, a company executive needed to be admitted to his local hospital for an emergency hernia repair. He looked after his health and paid attention to reported quality indicators across different businesses. He was well aware that his local hospital did not feature highly in the 'hospital league tables' and friends and colleagues reported mixed-views about their experiences with the hospital – unfriendly staff, inefficient systems, poor quality food and lack of information. So it was with a high degree of trepidation (and pain!) that he agreed to be taken to the hospital. However, his experience in the emergency department was nothing like those reported by others and to him did not reflect the league table score. He found staff to be friendly and courteous. They explained the 4-hour wait target in the emergency department and that they would do their best to have him admitted to a ward within that time-frame. He had a full assessment and was given analgesia to reduce the immediate pain. Within 2 hours David had surgery. His postoperative care was efficient and he felt that his medical care was well managed. He felt that the nursing care lacked continuity as different nurses undertook different tasks but he didn't feel that this impeded his care significantly as his priority was to be pain-free and leave hospital as quickly as possible. Overall, David was satisfied with his hospital experience and he began to question the value of global quality scores (such as league tables) compared with the actual experience in different parts of the hospital system.
>
> (personal communication, 2007)

How an idio-culture is experienced by staff and/or service users is dependent on the 'patterns' within the culture (Plsek, 2001). Plsek argues that within a workplace, patterns are associated with distinctive behavioural norms that manifest specific values, beliefs and assumptions, similar to Schein's levels of culture (Schein, 2004), where implicit emphasis is placed on how things are done and what counts as important. Plesk identified a number of patterns that shape workplaces, including:

- *decision-making:* rapid by experts versus hierarchy and position bound
- *relationships:* those that generate energy for new ideas versus those that drain energy
- *conflict:* existence of opportunities to embrace ideas versus the giving of negative and destructive feedback
- *power use:* power to enable versus power over
- *learning:* a culture where staff are eager to learn and improve versus experience of enforced learning that is threatening and risky to the status quo.

However, existing research into 'workplace climate' (the culture experienced by staff and service users) suggests that these patterns impact on productivity, job satisfaction, staff retention and organisational commitment, as well as individual perceptions of what it is like to work in their workplace (Tzeng, 2002; Slater, 2006). From our research underpinning the development of the PCN Framework, we identified characteristics of the workplace that are consistent with those identified by other authors as discussed here and as set out in Figure 5.1. It is these characteristics that the remainder of this chapter will address.

Points to Ponder

Have you ever thought about the culture of the place where you work? Do you think your workplace is similar or different to that espoused by the organisation? How would you describe the culture of your workplace?

Skill Mix

Debates about skill mix in nursing have existed throughout the history of nursing. Skill mix refers to the ration of registered (RNs) and non-registered nurses in a ward/unit nursing team. Skill mix is not a straightforward issue and in many ways the name is deceiving, that is it implies some kind of rational and logical relationship between the skills needed to undertake particular aspects of nursing work and the allocation of staff. In reality this is far from the case as skill mix management requires complex decisions of 'balance' to be made with regards to the nature of work undertaken (e.g. complexity and acuity), numbers of staff needed to provide a quality service and the skills and competencies of nurses to undertake the required work.

However, it is increasingly the case that skill mix decisions are driven by an economic agenda and the requirement of organisations to provide the most effective service at the lowest possible costs. As the drive for more cost-effective health services continues, the nursing workforce, as the largest part of a health service's workforce, is increasingly targeted, with the focus being on reducing the number of (expensive) RN hours and replacing those hours with (cheaper) non-registered staff hours. International analysis of nursing workforce trends demonstrates the consistent reduction of RN hours in many parts of the health care system and particularly in services that are not considered to be 'specialist' (Duffield et al., 2007). Interestingly, at the same time as the reduction in RN hours has been happening, health care policy increasingly places 'the provision of person-centred services' at the centre of policy and strategy developments (the National Service framework for Older People [DoH England] 2001a, 2007; European Commission, 2005). Thus, the question can be asked – is there any relationship between skill mix and PCN? Central to the answering of this question is consideration of the value placed on different kinds of nursing work.

> Joanna is a first year RN in an Intensive Care Unit (ICU). She works as a member of an all RN nursing team and provides 1:1 care on each of her shifts. As a new RN she has a mentor who work-shadowed her for the first 6-months in ICU and now 8 months into her post, she has an appointed supervisor/team leader who helps her plan her work on each shift and with her, evaluates the care delivered on each shift. She feels very privileged to be able to focus on 1 patient for each shift and understands why this is the case in an ICU (given the acuity of the patients she cares for and the instability of their health status). She values the time she has to focus on the 'non-technical' aspects of care, such as the provision of comfort measures, supporting families and 'being with' the patient and family. However, she reflects back on her last position as a third year student nurse on a surgical ward in the same hospital (specialised in colorectal surgery) where she regularly had six patients to care for on a morning shift and a 'good day' meant she got through the shift safely and without any major incidents happening. She often felt unsupported as the RNs focused on their patient case load and despite feeling that she was a valued member of the team, she regularly felt stressed by her work and dissatisfied that she was unable to work in the way she had been taught. She feels her work now in ICU is person-centred and wonders how she could have been more person-centred with patients on the surgical ward?

Nursing work has been characterised in a variety of ways – for example, technical versus non-technical; direct versus indirect; skilled versus unskilled; acute versus non-acute and urgent versus non-urgent. The majority of these categorisations are morally loaded terms suggesting a hierarchy of 'value or worth' placed on different activities, roles and functions that are undertaken by nurses of different grades, qualification and experience. So who or what determines the value or worth of nursing work?

The concept of 'worth' is complex. As was argued in Chapter 2, valuing personhood requires an adoption of a position that respects and values the intrinsic value of persons, that is persons are of value

Person-centred care is like an onion. I see the development of person-centred care as the unpeeling of different layers of the onion. Each time you peel off a layer (which may represent ritualistic care or non-person centred language) there is always another layer underneath to get stuck into. It takes resilience to get to the care and if you cut the onion in the wrong way – it makes you cry.

in and of themselves and should be respected as such. However, in an increasingly commercial world of health care, this moral ideal of personhood is constantly challenged. The worth of a health care intervention or treatment is often judged from an economic utilitarian perspective, that is the cost of the intervention balanced against the value (to society for example) of the outcomes achieved (Bowling, 2005). Increasingly in health care we see such decisions of economic worth creeping into health care decisions – the most often cited example being 'QALYS' (quality adjusted life years), which is a measure of 'payback', that is if a particular health care intervention (often surgical in nature) is performed, then over how many years would the value of that procedure be paid back to society (Prieto & Sacristán, 2003; Phillips & Thompson, 2009). Clearly this measure is controversial and morally loaded and is the subject of much debate in the health care literature (McGregor, 2003). Similarly, in the context of nursing work, the worth of the nursing input is considered alongside the assessed complexity of decision-making needed, the acuity of the care situation and the level of competency (usually technical competence) needed to undertake particular procedures. Thus, for example, intensive care units will have a significantly higher level of RNs compared with an aged care facility.

So what we come to understand is that those activities that are considered to be more technically complex (t), that require complex decision-making (d) and are linked to the degree of threat/risk (r) experienced by the patient are deemed to require more input from registered nurses. So decisions about skill mix are often calculated on the relationship between $t + d + r$. Whilst this relationship holds a high degree of logic and can be used to justify the need for education, training, specialisation and rates of pay in nursing in terms of the worth of nursing work, it places greater value on tangible, observable and objectively measurable activities. However, when service users are asked for feedback on the quality of services, the technical aspects of nursing work are often 'taken for granted' and feedback usually focuses on the more 'relationship'-oriented experiences, the provision of comfort and aesthetic experiences (Edwards et al., 2004; McCormack et al., 2008).

Equally seriously, reducing nursing work to tangible, observable and objectively measurable activities runs contrary to extensive evidence demonstrating the complexity and diversity of nursing work. In the United Kingdom, The Royal College of Nursing (RCN) describe nursing as:

> The use of clinical judgement in the provision of care to enable people to improve, maintain, or recover health, to cope with health problems, and to achieve the best possible quality of life, whatever their disease or disability, until death.

The RCN suggest that the defining characteristics of nursing are:

1. *A particular purpose:* the purpose of nursing is to promote health, healing, growth and development, and to prevent disease, illness,

injury and disability. When people become ill or disabled, the purpose of nursing is, in addition, to minimise distress and suffering, and to enable people to understand and cope with their disease or disability, its treatment and its consequences. When death is inevitable, the purpose of nursing is to maintain the best possible quality of life until its end.

2. *A particular mode* of intervention: nursing interventions are concerned with empowering people, and helping them to achieve, maintain or recover independence. Nursing is an intellectual, physical, emotional and moral process, which includes the identification of nursing needs; therapeutic interventions and personal care; information, education, advice and advocacy; and physical and emotional support. In addition to direct patient care, nursing practice includes management, teaching, policy and knowledge development.

3. *A particular domain:* the specific domain of nursing is people's unique responses to and experience of health, illness frailty, disability and health-related life events, in whatever environment or circumstances they find themselves. Human resources may be physiological, psychological, social, cultural or spiritual, and are often a combination of all of these. The term 'people' includes individuals of all ages, families and communities, throughout the entire life span.

4. *A particular focus:* the focus of nursing is the whole person and the human response rather than a particular aspect of the person or a particular pathological condition.

5. *A particular value base:* nursing is based on ethical values that respect the dignity, autonomy and uniqueness of human beings, the privileged nurse–patient relationship, and the acceptance of personal accountability for decisions and actions. These values are expressed in written codes of ethics, and supported by a system of professional regulation.

6. *A commitment to partnership:* nurses work in partnership with patients, their relatives and other carers, and in collaboration with others as members of a multidisciplinary team. Where appropriate they will lead the team, prescribing, delegating and supervising the work of others; at other times they will participate under the leadership of others. At all times, however, they remain personally and professionally accountable for their own decisions and actions.

(RCN, 2003: 3)

This articulation of nursing is consistent with the PCN Framework underpinning this book, that is, it articulates that there is a relationship between the attributes of the nurse, the environment in which nursing takes place, the activities undertaken by nurses and the resulting outcomes. This Framework extends nursing beyond that of providing technical care as the key consideration in the determination of skill mix and raises the issue of skill mix decisions extending beyond the tangible and objective aspects of work, thus reducing

To me you don't need a huge amount of resources to be person-centred and it is the small changes that matter. All you need is commitment, enthusiasm, a positive attitude and belief that the model will work no matter what environment you are in.

the potential for some client groups being deprived of access to registered nurses.

This has been an argument made by advocacy and professional groups on behalf of vulnerable populations (aged care, people with intellectual disabilities, people with physical disabilities in need of rehabilitation). Further work by the RCN with a particular focus on nursing older people in nursing homes articulated the differing knowledge, skills, expertise and role functions needed to be effective (RCN, 1996, 2004). Similarly, a recent guidance from the UK Nursing and Midwifery Council (NMC) (2009) highlights the important role of the registered nurse in delivering quality care that promotes dignity through the nurturing and supporting self-respect and self-worth among older people.

In a care home, registered nurses have multiple roles that reflect the diverse nature of nursing. Different functions that contribute to the optimum health and overall wellbeing of older people include:

- *Supportive* – including psychosocial and emotional support, assisting with easing transition, enhancing lifestyles and relationships, enabling life review, facilitating self-expression and ensuring cultural sensitivity.
- *Restorative* – aimed at maximising independence and functional ability, preventing further deterioration and/or disability, and enhancing quality of life. This is undertaken through a focus on rehabilitation that maximises the older person's potential for independence including assessment skills and undertaking essential care elements, for example, washing and dressing.
- *Educative* – the registered nurse teaches self-care activities – for example, self-medication – health promotion, continence promotion and health screening. With other staff, the registered nurse engages in a variety of teaching activities that are aimed at maximising confidence in competence and continuously improving the quality of care and service delivery.
- *Life*-enhancing – activities that are aimed at enhancing the daily living experience of older people, including relieving pain and suffering and ensuring adequate nutrition.
- *Managerial* – the registered nurse undertakes a range of administrative and supervisory responsibilities that call for the exercise of managerial skills. Such responsibilities include the supervision of care delivered by other staff and the overall management of the home environment.

Extract from 'Nursing Assessment and Older People: A Royal College of Nursing toolkit', Royal College of Nursing, London (2004: 6, 7).

How we determine skill mix does impact on the person-centredness of care processes. However, whilst much research has been undertaken into skill mix in nursing (Blegen, Goode & Reed, 1998; Spillsbury & Meyer, 2001; Estabrooks et al., 2005; Duffield et al., 2007), there are as yet few definitive models for determining skill mix.

In an evaluation of 11 outcomes that were determined to be sensitive to nursing intervention Duffield et al. (2007) determined a relationship between the available RN hours in medical and surgical wards and patient outcomes:

> A skill mix with a higher proportion of RNs produced statistically significant decreased rates of negative patient outcomes such as decubitus ulcers, gastrointestinal bleeding, sepsis, shock, physiologic/ metabolic derangement, pulmonary failure as well as 'failure to rescue'

> (Duffield et al., 2007: 16).

The authors identified that an extra RN shift per patient per day in the same settings would reduce the incidence of decubitus ulcers by 20 per 1000 patients; reduce the incidence of pneumonia by 16 per 1000 patients and reduce the incidence of sepsis by 8 per 1000 patients per day (p. 16). In addition, patients were less likely to fall and suffer an injury as RN hours increased, but falls with an injury increased when other nursing roles increased (such as enrolled nurses). Specialist nursing support, the presence of a nurse educator and a reduction in 'casual' nurses on a ward were associated with fewer medication errors. 'Nurses delaying the completion of tasks predicted increased rates of adverse events' (p. 17). In a review of the evidence influencing nurses 'intention to leave', Slater (2006) proposed a conceptual model that postulated relationships between key individual and organisational factors. One such factor was 'stress' and a key indicator of the existence of that factor was nursing skill mix, and that stress was associated with job-satisfaction and burnout. A consistent issue in determining the effectiveness of nursing is the issue of nursing autonomy and in particular the autonomy of nurses to engage in decisions about patient care.

Shared Decision-Making Systems

We have consistently reiterated the importance of person-centredness being about both patients/service users and staff. In this context it is essential that staff experience ways of engaging that facilitate active participation in decision-making and systems that support such decision-making in practice. Central to such a system is an effective team.

The essence of creating and sustaining a dynamic but strong; creative but stable; imaginative but grounded team is the paying attention to task, group and individual components in equal measures (Adair, 1987). Work in any one area (task, group or individual) will impact on the other two. So for example, if a particular task is managed well, the effects will impact on the group's learning for future task achievement and on individuals in terms of satisfaction, reward and development. Such a balance in teamwork is not achieved by 'chance' and requires considerable attention to and ongoing support for team building. This needs to be an integrated component of day-to-day teamwork. It requires a commitment to team relationships and processes.

Whilst one-off 'away days' are useful for taking stock, reviewing, consolidating and planning team objectives, systems, processes and relationships, they do not in themselves build an effective team.

Team building and team development needs to be an ongoing process and an integrated part of workplaces. The development of an effective person-centred and evidence-informed workplace requires the continued commitment to the development of a learning culture at work. Learning cultures are productive cultures, characterised by their ability to tolerate productive tensions, learn from mistakes, support and enable innovation, maximise individual potential and understand the interrelationship between team/system processes and the effectiveness of outcomes achieved (Titchen & Binnie, 1995; Kaye & Jordan-Evans, 2005). A learning culture is a culture where nurses view their work as exciting and revitalising offering them the prospect for both personal and professional growth. Creating an environment in which learning occurs takes account of the ward/unit atmosphere, the context within which nursing takes place (acute, community, etc.) and the process used to enable learning to occur.

Senge (2006) suggests that sustained learning only occurs in a supportive context and where learning is viewed as an integrated component of practice. Numerous studies have identified that investing in learning at work can develop the effectiveness of the workplace culture (Platzer et al., 2000; Clarke, 2001), facilitate an exciting workplace environment where challenge is part of everyday practice and ensure that learning extends beyond the boundaries of the clinical unit (Platzer et al., 2000). The key goal in the development of a positive learning culture is to recognise and overcome individual, group and organisational barriers in order to move towards an effective culture (Hoff et al., 2004) and overcome the features of workplaces that nurture horizontal violence.

In an action research study, Donna Brown worked with nursing teams in a surgical unit to develop the effectiveness of teamwork so as to improve the quality of pain assessment and management with older people. Donna identified there was a lack of:

- clarity around roles
- recognition of one another's skills and expertise
- value in individual roles
- clear leadership
- individual responsibility being taken by staff nurses.

A combination of role clarification, values clarification and continuous stakeholder evaluation were used to develop clarity of roles, maximise available skills and expertise and develop leadership potential. In addition, Donna engaged as a 'critical companion' (Titchen, 2004) with the leaders of the unit and worked through these issues in order to develop a culture of shared decision-making and collaborative working.

(Brown, 2008)

Continuous and integrated team building should include:

- ongoing values clarification
- clinical Supervision
- mentorship
- regular team meetings
- collaborative decision-making
- case review
- individual development plans/learning contracts
- reflective discussions
- conflict management
- critical evaluation.

Power Sharing and Effective Staff Relationships

Whatever approach to ongoing team development is chosen, the issue of power in teams is an inevitable issue and one that is important to consider when thinking about the development of shared decision-making and PCN. Power is a prevailing issue in society and our very existence requires the negotiation and renegotiation of power relationships. As Foucault (1982: 778) asserts '... *while the human subject is placed in relations of production and of significa-tion, he [sic] is equally placed in power relations which are very complex*'. Thus, it should be no surprise that power is an important issue in nursing and in the relationships between nurses and patients. As we have discussed earlier, the dominant view of nursing as an 'oppressed profession' is held almost unquestioningly among nurses and as Farrell (2001) argues, is often used too freely to explain abusive and power-driven relationships in nursing.

A simple historical critique of nursing though highlights the way in which power has dominated the discourse of nursing throughout its existence. Whilst Florence Nightingale may have considered her role to be one of 'service', accounts of Nightingale's modus operandi would suggest that she exerted power and influence in her daily work (Smith, 1982). Within nursing, individual power was invested in the matron and ward sisters. The hierarchical structures within which nursing operated meant that positional power was exerted freely by those 'in charge' and nursing staff had little control over their practice. The evolution of nursing through military and religious orders further reinforced the service discourse of nursing and the role of nurses to 'obey' those in senior positions. Further social and historical analysis has asserted that the dominant role of men in medicine and management has prevented nursing (predominantly female) from influencing outside of nursing.

Nursing has made considerable inroads in exerting power in health care decision-making and in shaping health care delivery politically and strategically. Western society in general, however, relies less on positional/hierarchical power and some argue that traditional theoretical perspectives of power do little to help understand the nature of power relationships in contemporary society. Foucault (1982) suggests that there are generally three types of struggles in power relationships:

1. The struggle against forms of domination: in nursing examples of domination might include, medical, management, religious, ideological.
2. The struggle against forms of exploitation which separate individuals from what they produce: in nursing examples of this exploitation might include task-orientated approaches to practice, hierarchical decision-making, allocation of unsocial hours unequally and non-payment of additional hours worked.
3. The struggle against subjection, that is the values that tie the individual to him/herself – in nursing examples of subjection might include the imposition of an organisation mission-statement without consultation, leaders insisting on approaches to practice that go against the shared values of a nursing team, rotation of nurses between departments thus preventing the establishment of meaningful relationships and a sense of security.

Foucault goes on to argue that there is a direct relationship between power and struggles against power (when seen as domination, exploitation or subjection):

> At any moment the relationship of power may become a confrontation of two adversaries. Equally, the relationship between adversaries in society may, at every moment, give place to the putting into operation of mechanisms of power (p. 794).

Foucault argues that a consequence of this scenario is the interpretation of the same relationship from different standpoints, either one of struggle or of power. Thus, it might be too easy to view nursing's history as a struggle against external power that dominated and controlled nurses and the practice of nursing. Indeed, Laverack (2005) argues that self-esteem is a key factor in exerting power and that for a profession to use power appropriately, it must have a strong sense of its own sense of self-worth. Laverack suggests three types of power, power-from-within, power-over and power-with. In a recent review of power theories, Bradbury-Jones et al. (2008) suggested that these types of power can be understood as self-esteem, domination and shared power. Both Laverack's (2005) and Bradbury-Jones et al. (2008) conceptualisations of power from nursing and health care perspectives help us to view power in a more positive light and to overcome the vagaries of power as articulated by Foucault.

Nursing has striven to move away from organisational systems that invoke domination, exploitation and subjection and has developed a greater self-esteem and confidence. However, Bradbury-Jones et al. argue that in order to facilitate the empowerment of others (a component of PCN) then nurses need to challenge existing practices that cause domination, move away from a reliance on hierarchical power/domination and understand the critical role of knowledge as power. Models of nursing derived from nursing theories (e.g. the Burford Nursing Development Unit Model of Nursing [Johns, 1994]; team nursing and primary nursing [Manthey, 2002]) can all be seen as significant developments in reshaping the nature of power relationships in nursing and challenging stereotypical hierarchical relationships.

Points to Ponder

Have you ever felt ridiculed or publically criticised at work? How did that make you feel? What did you do about it? Are you aware of such practices in your team? Think about the implications of these ways of engaging on others and on person-centredness in your workplace? What can you do to change this culture?

As a profession that predicates its foundations on 'caring', nursing has a checkered track record in terms of the demonstration of caring attributes in staff and team relationships. Many nurse theorists have conceptualised nursing as a caring profession. What is obvious from these different conceptualisations is that these theorists do not distinguish between caring in the context of patient care and caring in staff–staff relationships. Indeed, Boykin and Schoenhofer (1993) describe the 'dance of caring persons' as the fundamental basis of all caring relationships. They describe effective relationships as a 'dance' between persons, a dance that is seamless and synergistic with each dancer being responsive to the other in order to achieve mutuality.

However, the values of mutuality, collegiality and care that are espoused in mission statements and organisational frameworks are often not realised by staff in practice. Despite a large literature on teams, team effectiveness and team culture, dysfunctional team relationships continue to exist in nursing and health care (Cox, 2003; Wilson, 2005; Brown & McCormack, 2006).

Horizontal violence as negative power relationship

Defined as an act of aggression perpetrated by one colleague towards another colleague (Longo & Sherman, 2007), horizontal violence between nurses has been extensively documented. McKenna et al. (2002) suggest that the existence of horizontal violence in nursing is one of nursing's greatest paradoxes given its emphasis on caring and caring relationships. Horizontal violence rarely takes the form of physical aggression but instead is characterised by psychological harassment which creates hostility. This harassment is experienced through verbal abuse, threats, intimidation, humiliation, excessive criticism, innuendo, exclusion, denial of access of opportunity, disinterest, discouragement and the withholding of information (McKenna et al., 2002).

Sarah is a new nurse manager of a busy surgical ward. Prior to her appointment she was a staff nurse in the same unit. Sarah inherited a highly hierarchical culture from the previous nurse manager, who nobody openly criticised, but staff were generally discontented with her leadership. She was determined to change the culture of the unit and worked with the Directorate Practice Development (PD) facilitator to instigate a range of initiatives including, values clarification, team meetings, a new nursing model and a number of forums for staff to discuss and reflect on practice. However, the senior staff nurses ($n = 3$) (who had supported the previous nurse manager) did little to enable agreed ways of working to be fully realised. In her absence, they reverted to previous unit 'norms' and engaged in a variety of behaviours that staff disliked, ran contrary to agreed ways of working and undermined the vision that Sarah had for the unit. Some staff complained to her but did not want the senior nursing staff to know this as they were fearful of the consequences. Sarah met with the senior staff nurses to discuss what was happening and how they could work together to address the issues. The senior staff nurses would not recognise that there was a problem and suggested that she needed to be a 'stronger' leader and everything would be ok. In the subsequent weeks they commenced a 'whispering campaign', sowing seeds of doubt in the minds of other nurses, medical consultants and ancillary staff about Sarah's abilities as a leader and manager. Sarah knew it was happening but struggled to establish any evidence-base to prove it. She became disillusioned and cautious in her style and found it increasingly difficult to trust colleagues. The medical staff complained to the Directorate manager about problems on the ward and this further undermined her authority. A development programme was put in place to help develop her leadership. Whilst some things changed for the better and she regained some of her confidence, she resigned from her post after 12 months feeling stressed and disillusioned and vowing never to take up a leadership position again.

Farrell (1999) found that even though nurse–nurse aggression was not the type of aggression most often experienced or witnessed at work (doctor-to-nurse aggression was most often experienced/witnessed) it was nurse-to-nurse aggression that respondents cited as the most distressing to deal with. Adair (1987) suggests that an effective team may be defined as one that achieves its aim in the most efficient way and is then ready to take on more challenging tasks if so required. Adair suggests that an effective team has a particular focus that is known to all stakeholders (the task), pays attention to the needs of individuals in the team and continuously reviews team processes for their effectiveness. Whilst the existence of horizontal violence in teams is shown to undermine team effectiveness, Farrell (2001) suggests that little attention is given to understanding the causes of interpersonal conflict in nursing, other than by 'oppression theory'.

Nursing has been described as an oppressed group because it is predominantly a female occupation that has existed under a predominant patriarchal leadership, management and organisational system (Freshwater, 2000). Oppressed groups experience little autonomy or control over their work-life and as a consequence enter a cycle of low self-esteem and powerlessness. Oppressed groups experience frustration at their situation but feel powerless to address the circumstances of the oppression with superiors or the part of the system that is seen to cause the oppression, due to fear of retaliation or negative consequences (such as job loss). Instead, negative behaviours associated with the frustration is targeted at colleagues and they become the victim. In his classic study of the impact of imperial power on their colonies, Frantz Fanon (1967) suggests that oppressed groups engage in intergroup conflict as a means of releasing frustration that has built up because of the group's inability to attack the oppressor:

> But if the whole regime . . . are conditioned by a thousand year old oppression, your passivity serves to place you in the ranks of the oppressor . . .

Twenty years as a nurse
Moving through the ranks knowing who I am
Knowing me
Becoming a manager, being a manager
Managing
Discovering the joys of person-centredness
Unfurling the challenges of being a person-centred
leader
Self growth
Discovery
Transformation
The winds of change blow from the west
Person-centred leadership devalued
Targets
Bullying
Devaluing
I am an 'It'
Stats mean good care
Shared experiences mean coercion
Get out get out get out
Stay safe
Shut down
Hide
But I need to keep listening to the patients
    (Poem written by a Clinical Leader, 2008 [anonymous])

Fanon's work demonstrates the destructive impact of domination and suppression and the ways in which it erodes confidence among oppressed groups leading to internal conflict. This cycle of conflict becomes a self-fulfilling prophecy, that is, nurses cannot be trusted to manage themselves and so need to be managed by others, thus increasing the sense of frustration and oppression. Other explanations for horizontal violence include the self-effacing and masochistic nature of nursing, feelings of being 'abused' in nursing leading to increased hostility towards others, sex-role stereotyping, competitiveness and imbalance in power relationships (Farrell, 2001). However, Farrell goes on to argue that focusing on oppression as the only explanation for horizontal violence in nursing has resulted in a failure to explore other contributing factors. Farrell suggests that other causes of horizontal violence include:

- *Task/time imperatives*: the structuring of work according to time-based lists of tasks, that if uncompleted on time become a source of conflict.
- *Generational and hierarchical abuse*: socialisation into a culture of nurse–nurse abuse brought about by a belief that because the nurse in a senior position experienced horizontal violence she has a right to do the same to junior staff.
- *Clique formation*: exclusive identification with a sub-group and withdrawal of meaningful interaction with the larger group.
- *Low self-esteem*: negative comparison of evaluative outcomes of own group with those of other groups.
- *Aggression breeding aggression*: where aggression gets results its perpetrator is likely to be reinforced, thus continuing the likelihood of its existence.
- *Actor–observer effects*: viewing our behaviour as a consequence of factors beyond our control and the behaviour of others as a result of his/her personal dispositions.

These causes of horizontal violence are negative features of a workplace culture and Manley (2004) and others (Wilson et al., 2005; Brown, 2008) have demonstrated that a systematic approach to practice development can address these features and produce an effective workplace culture.

Potential for Innovation and Risk-Taking

There is no doubt that for PCN to exist, there is a need for a work organisation method that enables nurses to exercise power whilst simultaneously being able to negotiate the nature of that power in relationships with others (including patients and families). There is a large literature on empowerment and the essence of the power relationship between nurses and patients/families is the facilitation of empowerment. The language of empowerment is pervasive in nursing and contemporary nursing policy and strategy espouses the importance of nurses being empowered to exercise autonomous decisions, whilst at the same time empowering patients. Various authors have argued that the language of empowerment is complex and challenging, that nurses aren't empowered professionally or organisationally to exercise empowerment or to empower others (such as patients and families [Laschinger et al., 2000, 2001, 2003]).

It is our contention that nurses (nor indeed other health care workers) are in a position to empower others, but instead nurses can facilitate others to make empowered decisions and organisations need to create the conditions in which clinical staff are enabled to facilitate empowerment.

PCN makes explicit the need for nursing autonomy, equality in relationships and the centrality of beliefs and values in guiding decision-making. Contemporary work into the development of 'models of care' that have the patient at the centre and the nurse positioned to facilitate autonomous decision-making can be seen as attempts to re-orientate the design of health care services towards ones that are based on patient, family and staff experiences.

The New South Wales Health Department Models of Care Project

The Nursing Models of Care Project was established by the NSW Health Nursing and Midwifery Office in 2004 as a four-year program to assist clinical nurses to:

- explore and develop innovative models of nursing care delivery and organisation that would facilitate best clinical practice;
- develop new and emerging roles and partnerships within nursing and health care.

Workshops, seminars and roadshows have been a feature of the project, involving frontline nursing and midwifery staff and senior clinicians across NSW using their local experience and knowledge to help implement new models of care across the State.

http://www.health.nsw.gov.au/nursing/projects/
models_of_care.asp

In addition, the ongoing research into organisations known as 'Magnet Hospitals' has begun to illustrate the organisational conditions that are necessary for staff to feel empowered. Magnet hospitals have been associated with organisational attributes that have been positively linked to nursing staff outcomes (Aiken & Sloan, 1997a,b; Aiken et al., 1997). Magnet hospitals have specific organisational attributes that enable effectiveness of nursing practice and patient outcome. Their success is associated with three areas:

1. *Administration* – decentralised structures, flexible working, participatory and supportive management style, adequate staffing, the use of specialists and well-prepared and qualified nurse executives.
2. *Professional practice* – professional practice models of delivery, associated autonomy and responsibility, availability of specialist advice and emphasis on teaching.

3. *Professional development* – planned orientation of staff, emphasis on in-service/continuing education, competency-based clinical ladders and management development.

The findings from research by Aiken and colleagues reinforces the need for nurses to be recognised, supported and involved in decision-making about patient care and hospital governance through professional autonomy, an environment supportive of professional practice and development and strong supportive leadership (Gleason-Scott et al., 1999). 'Magnet' organisations enable professional nurses to use their knowledge and to do for patients what they know should be done in a manner consistent with their professional standards (Lewis & Matthews, 1998).

Tangible outcomes from Aiken's work include increased job satisfaction (Aiken & Fagin, 1997; Gleason-Scott et al., 1999; Upenieks, 2002), higher levels of recruitment and retention (McClure et al., 1983; Aiken & Fagin, 1997) even during periods of nurse shortage, increased quality of patient care (Kramer & Hafner, 1989; Aiken et al., 2001) and lower mortality and decreased time spent in hospital (Aiken et al., 1994). Aiken and colleagues conducted analysis into the organisational characteristics of hospitals with low turnover rates and low stress levels. They found that perceived level of autonomy was positively correlated with job satisfaction levels (Aiken, Clarke & Sloane, 2000; Finn, 2001), and associated with lower morality rates, better patient care as rated by the patients and better relationships with other health professionals (Aiken & Sochalski, 1997) across hospitals and within hospital wards. Blegen's international meta-analysis of studies into job satisfaction found that increased autonomy definitely contributes to increased job satisfaction (1993).

Professional autonomy is ranked as one of the most important factors contributing to nurses' job satisfaction (Stamp & Piedmonte, 1986). The researchers define autonomy as 'the amount of job independence, initiative, and freedom either permitted or required in daily work activities' (1986: 60). Autonomy is linked to clinical governance and accountability (Leddy & Pepper, 1993), and Manley (1996) argued that nursing professionalism hinges on autonomy. Despite the importance of autonomy, many nurses perceive their levels of autonomy to be limited (Oermann & Bixek, 1994). Two reasons have been given for this: (1) the overlap with other medical professionals, such as doctors has caused them to fail to believe in their rightful place alongside these health professionals, and (2) aggressive horizontal violence where nurses are oppressed by other nurses (usually higher grade) using the same autocratic principles that other health professionals use on them (Brown, 2008). Adherence to this method of personnel management is reflective of an outdated bureaucratic style of management.

In previous research, McCormack (2001a) suggested that for nurses to exercise their autonomy as a positive force in the enabling of effective quality care with patients, that there is a need to understand autonomy as 'interconnectedness'. The idea of autonomy as 'interconnectedness' is well established in the literature (Gilligan, 1982;

Gadow, 1990; Agich, 1993; Tronto, 1993) and is based on the premise that people are sometimes autonomous, sometimes dependent and sometimes provide care to those who are dependent (Tronto, 1993). Therefore, people are best described as 'interdependent'. Tronto argues that individualistic notions of 'autonomy as independence' places autonomy and dependence at either end of a continuum, but in reality, dependency in some aspects of life does not lead to dependency in all aspects of life.

McCormack (2001) argued that (from the perspective of older people services) the way such dependency is managed can lead to feelings of either hope and trust or despair and mistrust, as the older person attempts to accommodate the dependence associated with the incapacity as well as needing to rely on caregivers for help in dealing with the initial state of dependence. McCormack compared the data from registered nurses working in older people rehabilitation settings with the data of a community nurse specialist and a nationally recognised 'expert gerontological nurse' and concluded that nurses need to engage with four processes in an interconnected relationship with patients in order to facilitate adaptation and decision-making:

- The facilitation of decision-making through information sharing and the integration of new information into established perspectives and care practices.
- The recognition of the importance of individual values on decision-making and of knowing how each person's values influence decisions made.
- The making explicit of intentions and motivations for action and the boundaries within which care decisions are set.
- The creation of a culture of care that values the views of the patient as a legitimate basis for decision-making whilst recognising that the (older) person does not always need to be the final arbiter of decisions.

Engaging with these processes can enhance the experience of decisional autonomy (autonomy over decisions made) even if the person's capacity for executional autonomy (ability to autonomously act on a decision) is limited.

Deborah, aged 19, has sustained a serious head injury in a road-traffic accident. She has recently recovered from the acute phase of her trauma and is now in a neuro-rehabilitation unit. She is making a steady recovery and day by day is able to engage in increasing levels of self-care. Deborah, however, still depends on the nursing and care staff to assist with most of her activities of daily living (ADLs). Whilst she has some periods of memory loss, on the whole, Deborah is fully able to participate in decisions about her care and treatment. Whilst her mother is very relieved that Deborah is making such a rapid recovery, she gets frustrated with Deborah's insistence on pushing herself more and more. Deborah's friends visit her and

(Continued)

request the nurses if they could take Deborah out in the car to a local park for coffee. The nurses in discussion with other members of the multidisciplinary team feel that this is appropriate. However, Deborah's mother is horrified at this request and insists that the nurses prevent this from happening. The nurses convene a meeting between Deborah and her mother. They are both highly emotional about the decision – Deborah gets angry at her mother and her mother becomes defensive and upset. The nursing staff can see that both Deborah and her mother have valid concerns and relay these back to them both to help them understand each other's perspective. Eventually they understand each other and a negotiated position is agreed, whereby Deborah would begin by having a short trip to a café with her mum and accompanied by her nurse, with the agreement, that if all went smoothly then Deborah would be able to go out with her friends.

Understanding autonomy from an interconnected as opposed to an individualistic perspective is important in the context of contemporary health care and PCN. At no time in the history of nursing has 'health care safety' been given more priority in strategic planning, effectiveness monitoring, quality improvement systems and accreditation programmes. Whilst at first it may seem that the relationship between person-centredness and working within 'risk-averse' health care systems is paradoxical, in reality, these two concepts are closely linked. Nieva and Sorra (2003) suggests that the safety of an organisation is the product of individual and group values, attitudes, perceptions, competencies and patterns of behaviour that determine the commitment to, and the style and proficiency of, an organisation's health and safety management. Organisations with a positive safety culture are characterised by communications founded on mutual trust, by shared perceptions of the importance of safety and by confidence in the efficacy of preventative measures. Thus, instead of 'patient safety' being driven by a set of rules and regulations, Nieva and Sorra propose a way of thinking about safety that places emphasis on culture, relationships, values, communication and professional autonomy. International health care developments and modernisation reforms all place emphasis on clinical and corporate governance, risk management/minimisation and patient safety. Internationally for nurses, codes of professional conduct act as the Framework within which professional nursing practice is ethically managed. For example in the United Kingdom, the Nursing and Midwifery Council (NMC) 'Code of Professional Conduct' http://www.nmc-uk.org/aArticle.aspx?ArticleID=3056 expects the highest ethical standards of nursing through adherence to agreed evidence-based standards, protocols and procedures and the exercising of professional accountability. However, the code also balances the need for such safe practice with respecting the patient as an individual, with individual needs, wants and desires (Figure 5.2).

As a registered nurse, midwife or specialist community public health nurse, you must respect the patient or client as an individual:

You must recognize and respect the role of patients and clients as partners in their care and the contribution they can make to it. This involves identifying their preferences regarding care and respecting these within the limits of professional practice, existing legislation, resources and the goals of the therapeutic relationship

(Nursing & Midwifery Council (2004) The NMC code of professional conduct: standards for conduct, performance and ethics.)

Figure 5.2 Excerpt from NMC code of professional conduct.

Thus exercising professional accountability is not set within a strict and rigid framework, but reflects the need to balance best available evidence with professional judgement, local information (such as audit data), professional opinion (where there is consensus of opinion) and patient preferences (Rycroft-Malone et al., 2004).

Immanuel Kant provides a useful way of thinking about this 'balance' when he outlines the differences between 'perfect and imperfect duties' (Sullivan, 1990). Perfect duties are strict and enforceable principles that can be 'forced' to honour the duty prescribed. Being moral entails compliance with valid rights, no matter whether doing so conflicts with other moral goods or other values.

In contrast, imperfect duties are *'wide, broad and limited' – 'they leave us a play-room for free choice in following the law' (Sullivan, 1990: 52)* as there is no means of offering an exhaustive and a priori account of how the duties are to be fulfilled. Such duties as compassion, concern, benevolence, respect and care would all be imperfect duties. One cannot force someone to be caring. Instead, imperfect duties rely on the moral character of the individual, or what Kitson (1987) refers to as *'a moral attitude'*. Kant views such duties as 'imperfect' because in clinical decision-making one may have to decide between competing duties, and account must be taken of the context in which decisions are made. So whilst the 'best' evidence may indicate a particular way of practicing, a patient's preference may not be for this course of action. A nurse, working in a person-centred way and exercising his/her accountability will balance the degree of risk involved in supporting patient preference, negotiate a way forward and be able to justify the final decision made. Thus, nurses should not only focus on developing reasoning and decision-making skills, but also on developing sensitivity and an individual sense of moral responsibility. In this sense, the importance of education for moral-reasoning and for the character traits that are desired in a relationship such as that between a nurse and patient is paramount. The complex relationship between nurses, patients, their families and other health care workers as well as the complexity of health and social care decision-making and internal and external constraining factors prevent a rigid approach to decision-making and the invoking of a risk-adverse culture of practice.

The Physical Environment

> . . . a beautiful health care unit is not necessarily one in which patients feel nurtured and supported. A patient who is frightened, lonely, and isolated from family and friends is not likely to notice the carefully decorated surroundings. It is only when the architecture and interior design works in concert with other . . . components that the environment can help a caring staff help a patient feel less lonely and isolated.
>
> (Arneill & Frasca-Beaulieu, 2003)

The physical environment of care has for a long time been recognised as having a significant impact on the care experiences and patient outcomes. Indeed Florence Nightingale placed a major emphasis on the quality and cleanliness of the environment and viewed this as being critical to patient recovery. However, as Arneill and Frasca-Beaulieu assert, the physical environment needs to work in concert with the cultural values in care teams and the ways of working that enable person-centredness to be realised. In this respect, two aspects of the physical environment need to be paid attention to – (1) the built environment; (2) the aesthetic environment.

The design of hospital wards/departments and other care facilities have changed significantly over the years. Research continues to demonstrate the important relationship that exists between the physical and sensory environment, health care outcomes and quality of life (for patients/residents and staff). There is now a wide evidence-base demonstrating the importance of the physical environment to care and healing. One of these significant developments has been the work of the 'Planetree Model' developed in 1978 (Frampton et al., 2003). The Planetree initiative set out to redress what was considered to be a reclaiming of holistic, patient-centred medicine and health care. Whilst the individual elements of the Planetree model reflect the PCN Framework a significant component of the Planetree model from the outset was the 'humanising' of the care environment. The model emphasised the importance of the care environment:

- welcoming the patient's family and friends
- valuing human beings over technology
- enabling patients to fully participate as partners in their care
- providing flexibility to personalise the care of each patient
- encouraging caregivers to be responsive to patients
- fostering a connection to nature and beauty.

Throughout the history of Planetree, these principles have been translated into a variety of health care settings, including emergency and intensive care departments, obstetric departments, medical/surgical units and outpatient facilities, as well as across whole hospitals (Arneill & Frasca-Beaulieu, 2003).

Whilst such programmes as the Planetree are exciting examples of the potential to change the environment of health care and capitalise on the potential of the environment to contribute to healing, the reality is that the majority of health care settings continue to be clinical, drab, depressing and soulless. Most hospitals and health care facilities have been designed with 'clinical efficiency' in mind and not person-centredness. However, considerable efforts are being made to ensure that new health care facility designs adopt a person-centred approach. But not all patients and staff can expect to work in facilities that are designed with person-centredness explicitly in mind and so there is a need to consider how existing environments can be enhanced. In one such initiative, the King's Fund developed the 'Enhancing the Healing Environment Programme'. An evaluation of the initial funded programme (Lowson et al., 2006) demonstrated both therapeutic and economic benefits, as well as positive experiences among participants. Other developments such as those of the 'Hospice friendly Hospitals Programme' in the Republic of Ireland draw upon 'evidence-based design' principles – 'a process-based approach to design that uses current best evidence from research and practice to create health care environments that improve patient and staff outcomes and operational performance' (Hospice friendly Hospitals, 2008). The guidelines developed are based on principles of dignity, privacy, sanctuary, choice/control, safety and universal access.

> The Enhancing the Healing Environment (EHE) programme encourages and enables nurse-led teams to work in partnership with patients to improve the environment in which they deliver care. It consists of two main elements:
>
> - a development programme for a multidisciplinary team, led by a nurse and including estates and facilities staff, arts co-ordinators, patients and strategic health authority representatives
> - a grant for the team to undertake a project to improve the patient environment.
>
> http://www.kingsfund.org.uk/research/projects/enhancing_the_
> healing_environment/approach.html

Similar design initiatives have occurred in residential care settings, particularly for older people and people with a dementia. The emphasis in these design developments has been on creating 'homes' that maximise the autonomy and independence of older people and people with a dementia, as well as ensuring the same principles as the Hospice friendly Hospitals Programme (dignity, privacy, sanctuary, choice/control, safety and universal access). Contemporary care homes aim to be more reflective of a home environment and focus on an overall 'domestic style', including, open plan kitchen/dining/living space; single ensuite rooms with personal belongings and furniture and reduction of obvious 'hospital-like' structures such as nurses stations (Dementia Services Development Centre, 2007; Kane et al., 2007).

Wagner's (1994) research into the normalising of care environments for older people is an example of an influential programme of work that has informed the design of care homes since the 1980s. In 1984 Wagner, a public health nurse, initiated a programme of work informed by participatory action research, to integrate the health and social care needs of older people with primary care principles. The programme of work that ensued resulted in large-scale de-institutionalisation of care homes/residential care facilities and a programme of social reform in residential care that has influenced residential care provision internationally. Known as the 'Skaevinge Project', the programme of work had person-centred principles at the core of its work and central to care home design and the care delivery model. Since then, the 'household' approach to care home design and care delivery has been growing in influence. With its roots in a belief that residential care homes should mimic 'normal homes' the household model attempts to de-institutionalise care homes. Such de-institutionalisation places emphasis on the importance of the kitchen and dining space in a home as a place of congregation, connection, nourishment and relaxation; the creation of spaces that nourish the human 'curiosity' (e.g. the organising of rooms and shared spaces to maximise opportunities to 'people watch'); the isolation of 'clinical activities' from everyday living activities and the reduction of the clinical artefacts of care (such as nurses stations, notice boards, treatment areas and drug trolleys); the separation of living and sleeping spaces (residents' rooms being in a separate space from communal and shared spaces) and the maximising of opportunities to engage with nature and outside spaces. Findings from research of this type of model suggest that older people have a better quality of life and improved functional status when compared with traditional models. Evidence has also shown that staff like to work in this way and significantly improved retention rates of staff have been recorded (Wagner, 1994; Kane et al., 2007).

The aesthetic environment is also a key consideration. Considerable developments have taken place in ensuring the environments are aesthetically pleasing and promote healing, nurturing, care, belonging and sensory engagement. The connection of the arts and humanities with health has been a major development in contemporary health care and is a significant movement internationally. The strategic placement of art (pictures, sculptures and instillations) for sensory and emotional stimulation; the use of different light, sounds and smells to promote relaxation and as therapeutic engagement and the integration of performance art with health care practice have all become more commonplace. Evidence from maternity services (Chang et al., 2008), people with dementia (Hannemann, 2006) and people with head injuries (Elliott, 2008) all demonstrate the positive therapeutic effect of integrated arts and health approaches. Examples of good practice in this field include the Northern Irish Charity 'Arts Care' http://www.artscare.co.uk/; the Kings Fund London programme of work aimed at enhancing the healing environment http://www.kingsfund.org.uk/; the Nuffield Trust arts and humanities programme http://www.nuffieldtrust.org.uk/; the London Arts in Health Forum http://www.lahf.com/welcome; the Arts Health Network Canada http://www.artshealthnetworkcanada.com/links/index.html and the Centre for Arts and Humanities in Health and Medicine, Durham University http://www.dur.ac.uk/cmh/.

Whatever the intent, be it therapeutic or social engagement, it is clear that in contemporary health and social care systems, aesthetics matter and the arts play a significant role in creating aesthetically pleasing spaces. Consistent with the ideas of space, place, body and time (Merleau-Ponty, 1989) articulated in Chapter 2, there is a direct relationship between the built environment and person-centredness. The structures and aesthetic qualities of the care environment are interconnected with an individuals' sense of self, sense of being and sense of connection with the world and as such are key considerations in the delivery of PCN.

Points to Ponder

Have you ever stopped and explored the physical environment in which you work? Try to find a time in a day when you could meaningfully walk around the environment asking yourself the following questions:

   What do I see?

   What do I hear?

   What do I feel?

   What do I smell?

   Think about the answers to these questions in the context of what it might feel like to be a patient or resident in that environment and how it enables (or not) dignity, privacy, sanctuary, choice/control, safety and universal access.

Summary of Key Points

This chapter has explored the care environment in the context of PCN. The chapter adopted the position that the characteristics of the care environment have the greatest potential to enhance or hinder PCN. Too often the care environment is treated as a malleable 'thing' that can be manipulated to suit rapid changing macro-health care contexts. The reality is that care environments are comprised of layers of cultures and characteristics that interact with each other, creating a complex weave of perspectives, relationships and behaviours. These layers and characteristics cannot be ignored when thinking about person-centredness and to suggest that person-centred relationships with patients can be formed without addressing these issues would be naïve and potentially harmful to staff and patients. So, current strategic agendas of patient safety and risk minimisation cannot be addressed in isolation and have to be explored and developed alongside developments of care environments that enhance person-centredness.

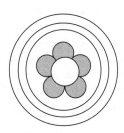

Chapter 6

Person-Centred Processes

Introduction

The previous two chapters have set the scene in terms of the attributes of the nurse and the elements within the care environment that enable the delivery of effective person-centred processes. In this chapter we will explore person-centred processes, which focus on delivering care through a range of activities that operationalise PCN. This is the construct within the Framework that specifically focuses on the patient, describing PCN in the context of care delivery (McCormack & McCance, 2006). In the original framework the following five components were presented: working with patient's beliefs and values; engagement; having sympathetic presence; sharing decision-making and providing for physical needs.

As highlighted in the introductory chapter the component focusing on 'providing for physical needs' has been revised as a direct result of feedback obtained through continuous testing in practice. Within the Framework we now use the term 'providing holistic care' in order to reflect not only the provision of physical aspects of care, but also the range of psychological, social, cultural and spiritual needs expressed by patients. The five components of the PCN Framework are presented in Figure 6.1 and will be used to structure this chapter. As is the case with previous constructs within the Framework, the person-centred processes are not mutually exclusive, but are often interwoven in the delivery of patient care.

Figure 6.1 Person-centred processes.

- working with patients' beliefs and values
- shared decision-making
- engagement
- having sympathetic presence
- providing holistic care

Working with Patients' Beliefs and Values

Working with patients' beliefs and values reinforces one of the fundamental principles of PCN, which places importance on

If you get to the roots of the plant and nourish them, it will keep on growing after it has been cut down. The small person becomes a big person.

developing a clear picture of what the patient values about his/her life and how he/she makes sense of what is happening. Reality refers to the everyday world and is imbued with personal meanings, beliefs and values that are essential to the way the person 'sees' themselves and the way their world is constructed. Whilst many aspects of an individual's reality may be shared with others so that common understandings can exist in order to form a sense of community, it is the individuality of our personal meanings that determines 'who I am'. In a nursing context, Gilligan (1982) suggests that a patient's true potential can be fulfilled if there is an attachment between the nurse and the patient that is based on the patient's unique value system. For Gilligan, each person is immersed in a web of ongoing relationships and being 'in relation' to another is a fundamental part of human existence.

Persons are defined by their historical connections and relationships requiring the nurse to take into account the particular person that the patient is, the particular relationship that exists between them and the patient, and the particular understandings and expectations implicit in the relationship (Blum, 1982). The nurse knowing about another's values and beliefs requires caring about the other in a way that appreciates an understanding of each patient as an individual human being. Such a particular caring knowledge of patients is necessary in order to determine a particular course of action to take from a variety of potential options. Merely applying a universal principle such as 'do no harm' (UKCC, 1992) or 'do not tell lies' does not inform the nurse what 'harm' means to the particular patient in the particular situation, thus inferring the need to get to know the patient. Clarke (2000) provides a very powerful example from a nurse who described how a patient used to get out of bed and wander around the ward at 4.00 a.m. every morning, which was initially labelled as confusion, only to discover that this patient was in fact a retired miner and had been used to getting up at this time every morning to go to work. Ericson et al. (2001), whilst acknowledging the importance of intimate knowledge of the person with dementia from the perspective of their carers, highlights the challenge for practitioners in obtaining the often 'implicit and subtle understanding of the views of the other' (p. 711).

The use of a biographical approach or life stories (see Chapter 2) is being promoted in the literature, particularly within care of older people (Clarke, 2000; McCormack, 2002) as a way of learning more about the patient as an individual. A person's biography can be seen as an account of a number of separate, but related life events that have influenced and directed the person's life. It is the history that gives meaning to the values of the individual and provides the explanations which are needed when crises occur and care decisions are being chosen (Johnson, 1991). Indeed Schofield (1994) suggests that an experienced nurse will be able to recognise when biographical details are important to clarify concerns in care, thereby identifying the appropriate focus of care and the maintenance of the person's integrity. Furthermore, the goal of a biographical approach is to uncover the rich diversity of people's lives, with the aim of reducing one's tendency to generalise based on one's own previous experience and pre-conceptions. Clarke et al. (2003) evaluated the introduction of a biographical approach to care on a unit in an NHS hospital within the United Kingdom mainly from the perspective of the practitioners who used it. The main findings indicated that using this approach encouraged practitioners to see the person behind the patient, and also helped build relationships with patients and their relatives. Interestingly, participants in Clarke et al.'s (2003) study felt that this approach would not be suitable for all patients and cites the example of those patients who would be more reserved and liked to maintain their privacy. This brings us back to the original premise of this element of the Framework – the need to understand what is important to the patient in order to be able to integrate personalised information into a plan of care. The following is an example pro-vided by a nurse during supervision where she is trying to balance taking risks and her professional accountability based on what she knows is important to the patient.

Sam came to us for several years for respite care. He enjoyed his daily whisky and always slept in his chair at night. He commented one day 'If I die tomorrow I'll be a happy man. I've had my time.' On this admission he was terminally ill and a pressure relieving mattress was prepared for him. He was restless and uncomfortable and determined to sleep in his chair. The look of relief on his face when we hoisted him out of his bed said it all. Whilst dying, we respected his wish for whisky and water. When he was unable to take oral fluids he had 'whisky-based mouth care'. He wasn't swallowing at the time and this was performed by his family. Sam's dignity was respected by letting him die in his chair with family and his whisky nearby. Immediately before his death, he swallowed some whisky from a sponge as if in a celebration, before dying shortly afterwards. Sam was a large man. I realised when I hoisted him into his chair that he would die there. This was important to him. When well he wasn't worried about his pressure relief or hygiene. These values are important to me but it would have been wrong to enforce these val-ues on to him. A pressure relieving cushion, however, was put in the chair. He wasn't moved from his chair for two and a half days. The first day we respected his wish not to be hoisted for pressure relief as he was in control of his care and said he was tired and wanted to rest. The second day it would have been totally inappropriate as he was far too ill and who would I be pleasing Sam or myself? I feel as long as I can account for my actions I made the right decision. Sam died without pain and without enforced nursing care.
(The story is derived from an account shared with Brendan during a Clinical Supervision session.)

The biographical approach is essentially about life stories and whilst this may be appropriate for care of older people, particularly in the context of making decisions that can result in major life changes, there is an argument that approaches need to be developed that enables nurses to obtain information about any patient. The focus should be on how their health problems impact on their life to ensure each individual can receive care that uniquely meets their needs. A person-centred assessment is key to obtaining information that builds up a picture of a patient as an individual with a unique life story. Webster (2004) discusses the challenges of person-centred assessment, in the context of older people, and identified factors that can contribute to an unsatisfactory approach to assessment such as: lack of involvement by the person to whom the assessment relates; limited skills, knowledge and experience in the person carrying out the assessment; adhering to rigid/unbending frameworks or tools for assessment; task focus or ritualistic practice and lack of connection between the assessment process and the ongoing care planning and evaluation. We would argue these factors are widely applicable to the family of nursing irrespective of the client group. Furthermore, this issue is also closely connected to the use of models or frameworks that underpin the assessment process, and to the thorny issue of nursing documentation. The risk is that the underlying assumptions and values of any model, if not given full consideration, can negatively impact on the care received by patients. Johns (1991) further argues that the structured nature of the assessment criteria derived from models can lead to assessment seen as a task to be completed. It is often specific criteria that direct the dialogue between a nurse and a newly admitted patient as opposed to engagement in a process that facilitates the gathering of information that begins to build up a picture of that patient as a person, which is illustrated by the following story.

Jack was a 41-year-old man who was admitted to an acute surgical ward for removal of a cancerous tumour. He arrived on the ward with his wife and was warmly welcomed and shown to his bed. A short time later a young nurse appeared and introduced herself as Maria and informed Jack that she was going to admit him. She proceeded to ask Jack a series of questions meticulously working her way through various forms, ticking boxes relating to previous medical history, current medications, eating habits, lifestyle issues such as smoking, exercise and so on. Maria was warm and engaging throughout and once she had completed all the relevant documentation she checked that Jack didn't need anything else and went on her way satisfied that she had done the job. What Maria, however, had failed to establish was how Jack felt about his diagnosis of cancer, how he felt about his planned surgery, what he was most anxious about and how he felt about leaving his two young children at home to come into hospital? The information Maria had gleaned during nursing assessment was useful to a point, but failed to provide a picture of Jack and what was important to him in his life, which needed to be integrated into his plan of care.

McCormack (2003) was able to make a link between the expertise of the nurse and the nurse's ability to glean and interpret information. More inexperienced nurses were seen to dismiss stories as irrelevant to the conversation or treat them as stories, that is, as fictional tales that had little relevance to the particular interaction. In contrast both the expert nurse and clinical nurse specialist were seen to adopt a differing approach and integrated patients' stories into the conversation, utilising their interpretations of stories to evaluate previous comments and formulate next questions. The second approach, the one that has greatest relevance to the facilitation of an individual's authentic consciousness, is an understanding of biography as an interpretative process. Agich (1993) is critical of technical approaches to biography and he argues that the uniqueness and individuality of stories is often overlooked. Life stories are not constructions of a past that is 'out there', separate from the individual's current experiences and that has been discovered through the process of storytelling. Instead, constructing a biography is an interpretative process that involves the conferring of meaning about oneself and the whole of one's life course. The purpose of the story is to make sense of the present in light of the past. Whether the account is objective or a subjective construction of a reality is not important, as it is the account developed in the present with the purpose of making sense of things.

Like the colour green, my experience of developing person-centred nursing represents a fresh new beginning. If a person feels that what they are doing is worthwhile and it matters, it filters to everyone and reflects everything that we do:

Work is a chore
Work is a bore
Choose an Angel
Feel its glow
Feel a colour
Let the feeling flow
Open our minds
Everything matters

Shared Decision-Making

This element of the Framework focuses on nurses facilitating patient participation in decision-making through providing information and integrating newly formed perspectives into established practices. It is closely linked to working with patient's beliefs and values and must involve a process of negotiation that takes account of individual values to form a legitimate basis for decision-making, the success of which rests on successful processes of communication (McCormack & McCance, 2006). There is a large and diverse literature about decision-making in professional practice. The focus, however, within the Framework is on how nurses can facilitate participation in shared decision-making that is underpinned by the principles of person-centredness. In Chapter 2 we identified that the right to 'self-determination' is a valued human right. If we do value self-determination, then it follows that we have the right to participate in decision-making about treatment, care options and processes. Drawing on the work of Gadow (1980), person-centred decision-making is based on the formation of an interdependent and interconnected relationship of persons and the belief that most health care decisions require a sharing of beliefs, values, perspectives and views between staff and patients:

> individuals [should] be assisted by nursing to authentically exercise their freedom of self-determination. By authentic is meant a way of reaching decisions which are truly one's own-decisions that express all that one believes important about oneself and the world, the entire complexity of one's values.

To work in this way requires a connectedness (Gilligan, 1982) between the nurse and the patient and a consideration of the patient as a whole person. McCormack (2001b) suggested that each interaction between a patient/family and a nurse denotes a 'care situation':

> The care situation focuses on the facilitation of a person's decision-making through the consideration of his or her values, experiences, moral principles and concerns. If each care situation is approached as a unique interaction and that the focus is on the interaction with *that* patient at *that* time, then ethical standards can be maintained based on the individual's life plan, with broader political factors acting as influences rather than controls (p. 260).

Person-centred decision-making holds central the knowledge and experience that each person brings to the care situation, which is necessary for decisions that will best serve the patient's well-being. Examples of this in the United Kingdom include, unified assessment schemes such as that in Northern Ireland (http://www.dhsspsni.gov .uk/ec-northern-ireland-single-assessment-tool-and-guidance) models for involving older people with dementia in decision-making (Dewing, 2002) and the expert–patient programme (DH, 2001b). At the heart of this style of nursing is the therapeutic nurse–patient relationship that requires continuity of care and the acceptance of responsibility for the outcomes of care. The aim is to transform the person's experience and enable them to consider a variety of perspectives that can help shape perceptions and understandings. The role of the person-centred nurse is to *be there*, offering personal support and practical expertise, whilst enabling the patient to follow the path of their own choosing and in their own way.

McCormack (2003) identifies mutuality as central to the process of shared decision-making, which recognises the others' values as being of equal importance in decision-making. A good nurse–patient relationship establishes a personal–professional connection based on mutual respect and honesty (Genevay & Katz, 1990). It involves 'being with' and 'doing with', through the active participation of the patient in order to activate the potential within themselves. If a nurse can trust in the relationship she has with a patient, then it is all right to be led by the patient, not in a passive sense of being led, but in a dynamic sense where the cues and nuances of the patient's behaviour direct the focus of the action that needs to be taken. The patient is thus given a real part to play in helping the nurse discover new ways of working and a real partnership is established. There are of course other times when firmness in approach has to be taken and sometimes without this firmness the person would feel insecure and at risk. However, as long as the reasons for this are negotiated into the plan of care, partnership can still be maintained. Through mutuality, those who care and those who are cared for, don't have to relate to each other as strong and weak, but both can grow in each other's capacity to learn from each other as equals.

Respecting the individual beliefs and value of the patient rejects the concept of paternalism and makes way for a model of decision-making based on the patient's value history. In collaborative decision-making, the nurse does not see herself as being in charge, but places the patient's values (or their advocate) central in determining a resolution in important decisions. The central tenet of the relationship is honesty and is influenced by communication skills, knowledge and experience of the patient, the patient's knowledge and experience, the patient's personality, the nature of the problem and the time available for the decision to be made. Whilst certain approaches may be more appropriate than others in particular cases, it is the individuality of the particular case that determines the way forward. For this reason, decision-making ought to take a joint approach between practitioner and patient, as each brings knowledge and experience that the other lacks, yet which is necessary for decisions that will best serve the patient's well-being (Buchanan & Brock, 1989: 30):

> In the exercise of their right to give informed consent, then, patients commonly decide in ways that they believe will best promote their well-being as they conceive it.

The adoption, however, of a passive role by a patient, that is a patient who does not want to participate in decision-making but expects the nurse to make the decision on their behalf, does not equate to a lack of autonomy, but instead is a confirmation of the patient's autonomy based on his or her values. Professional carers need to be open to listening and hearing patients stories and valuing this activity as an important part of care giving (Goldsmith, 1996; McCormack, 2002).

The need for the nurse to possess the necessary skills, however, to engage in shared decision-making and the potential impact of the care environment paints a complex picture. In McCormack's original study the findings indicated that many nurses adopted a position of 'information giving' as their dominant mode of operation. Their focus was that of providing information as a part of their commitment to patient participation. However, the lack of a clear framework in which such information was contained and the dominant role of professionals in decision-making, resulted in information acting as another form of control that served to reinforce decisions already made by professionals, rather than a means of enabling decision-making by patients themselves. The conversational style of nurses, including their control of the conversation agenda and the conversation focus, prevented patients from determining care outcomes for themselves. Nurses were clearly at an advantage over patients, because of their ability to identify salient features of conversations and integrate these into their already established 'picture' of the patient. In addition, it has been identified that patients have a limited understanding of the health care system compared to that of health care professionals, a further factor that places nursing staff at an advantage over patients.

Furthermore, basing care decisions on the patient's value history could be deemed idealist placing the nurse in a powerless position, whereby only those decisions that are made by the patient and that are consistent with their value history could be followed. Indeed it is argued (Fulford, 1996) that such a position reduces (nursing) to responding to the requests and demands of patients without a need to consider broader professional and sociological implications. In reality, however, many cases could be constructed where the patient may not be the best judge of their own well-being, for example the older person who insists on returning to their own home even though it is uninhabitable or an ill patient refusing life-saving treatment. Cases such as these do not present a sufficient argument for paternalistic decision-making by nurses. In collaborative decision-making, the nurse does not see herself as being in charge, but places the patient's values (or their advocate) central in determining a resolution in important decisions. Both patients' and nurses' values need to be respected in this kind of collaborative person-centred partnership and actively worked with in order to enable effective participatory decision-making to be realised.

Ann, a nurse specialist in diabetes is working with Ray and his wife. Ray has been treated with oral hypoglycemics for many years. However, his diabetes is becoming increasingly unstable and Ray's wife (Stella) reports that he is continuously sleepy, which Ann explains is probably due to high blood sugar levels. Ann is keen that Ray commences on insulin therapy. Ray is reluctant as he and his wife are nervous about the injection technique and how it would be managed. Ann explains: 'the reason I am trying to persuade you is that I have a really big feeling that you will feel so much more energetic, but it is really your choice, honestly'. Over a period of 2 weeks, Ann visited Ray and Stella and talked to them about the insulin regime, showed them different products, gave them leaflets and discussed their issues and concerns. Ann continuously emphasised that it was important that Ray and Stella make the choice once they had considered all the information provided. Ray and Stella made the decision to use insulin. The transparency in decision-making enabled Ann to balance her own accountability and values with those of the patient and his family.

Although the language of partnership is common place, it remains unusual for nurses to present their own views as a component of the array of information that patients are given to assist their decisions. Whilst the patient's values should be the decisive ones (Gadow, 1990) the nurse's values also contribute to the process. Indeed it could be argued that if a connected relationship exists between the nurse and patient, then it is especially important that the nurse's values are expressed – particularly when they conflict with the patient's values. If the nurse is truly working in partnership with the patient then there is no reason why the expression of such values should be coercive. Instead, the disclosure of the nurse's values may help the patient to understand particular approaches taken by the nurse and it may offer the patient an alternative view when considering their own values. In addition, the expression of values by the nurse serves to complete the partial perspective of the patient, with a focus that is formed from experience and knowledge of typical cases (Gadow, 1990). Such an approach, however, requires skilled and sensitive communication on the part of the nurse and an ability to judge when is the most appropriate time for disclosure. For example, it would be inappropriate to pre-judge a patient's partner as 'uncaring' should that person express the desire not to carry on a caring role. However, it may be appropriate to express the importance of family relationships as a means of helping the carer to see another perspective. Disclosure of values by the nurse is not to persuade the patient or inform them of most appropriate action. It is, however, as argued by Gadow (1990), a demonstration to the patient that the nurse considers values important not as a way of impersonally prescribing action, but as a professional commitment to ethical reflection. Johns (1999, 2005) reinforces the need for ethical reflection by the nurse as paramount in effective decision-making, which can also contribute to the development of clinical expertise (Hardy et al., 2006). A care environment that provides opportunities for clinicians to learn from their practice, explore and clarify their values and develop expertise in supporting patient-centred ethical decision-making, can enable the development of expertise in patient-centred practice (Titchen, 2009). These factors have been explored in Chapters 4 and 5.

Points to Ponder

Think of a recent experience when you were negotiating with a patient and their family regarding care options. How did you manage this process and what was the outcome? Can you describe your role in the decision-making process?

Engagement

Closely linked to shared decision-making is engagement, a process described in the PCN Framework as that which reflects the connectedness of a nurse with her/his patient. If we accept that each care situation is approached as a unique interaction and that the focus is on the interaction with *that* person at *that* time, based on their own values and beliefs we can assume the nurse is engaged with the patient. Benner and Wrubel (1989), however, would argue that total connectedness with a patient can lead to 'ethical blindness', and more realistically nurses will move between three 'stances' when working with patients, that represent different levels of engagement (connectedness) – full engagement, partial disengagement and complete disengagement (McCormack, 2003).

Full engagement is present when the patient and nurse are connected in the relationship and a care partnership exists. Collaborative decision-making takes place and the values of both nurse and patient are present at an unconscious level in the giving and receiving of care. The nurse may be aware of political, environmental and cultural pressures that affect the way she gives care, but she interprets and prioritises the salient features of such pressures and integrates these into her practice. A dilemma, however, may arise in the care relationship that affects the way the nurse and patient are able to work together. As a result *partial disengagement* occurs whilst the nurse takes stock of the situation and formulates the problem. At this point the interconnected working between the nurse and patient is interrupted, and whatever the cause, the relationship between the nurse and patient is altered and the nurse may lose the maximum grasp that was available whilst engaged with the patient (Benner & Wrubel, 1989). Such disengagement then requires a period of contemplation and, for a period of time, *complete disengagement* occurs. In this stance the nurse contemplates the available options from a more objective stance and re-assesses the values that underpin the relationship and decision-making. At this point the nurse needs to decide on appropriate action to reconnect the relationship. Support mechanisms such as reflective practice (Johns, 1998, 2005), clinical supervision (Bishop, 1998) and case reviews (Robbins, 1996) can help achieve this goal. Whilst the nurse continues to work with the patient in seeking the most satisfactory resolution, the connectedness in the relationship is broken until such time as a resolution can be found that is coherent with the values of the patient.

A skilled nurse will be able to adopt these three different stances at different times with the patient. Each stance may be short lived, but what is important is for the nurse to be able to move between these positions in order to stand back from the relationship with the patient, contemplate options and establish the most appropriate resolution. Having a clear picture of what the patient values about his life and how he makes sense of what is happening to him is needed, which provides a standard against which the practitioner can compare current decisions and behaviours of the patient.

Katrina was a nurse working in an acute mental health unit. She first met Michael when he was admitted to her unit and diagnosed with bipolar disorder, after experiencing symptoms of severe depression. Michael was married with three teenage children and had experienced suicidal intentions that contributed to high levels of distress for him and his family. Katrina became Michael's key worker and spent considerable time talking with Michael about his life and his experience of living with the symptoms of depression that influenced the onset of the suicidal thoughts and intentions he was struggling with. Katrina discussed the development of a programme of therapeutic intervention in partnership with Michael. The intention of this agreed programme was to promote Michael's recovery. During this time Katrina felt connected to Michael and his story about his experience and perceptions.

Michael, from the beginning, was reluctant to stay in the unit and was frequently very unsettled, desperate to get back home to his family. When Michael started feeling better his desire to get home increased even more and one day announced to Katrina that he felt well enough to be at home and wanted to discharge himself. Katrina, with many years of experience caring for people who were living with a bipolar disorder, felt that it was too soon to facilitate Michael's desire to be discharged. Katrina's anxiety was based on knowledge of his symptoms and the reduced protective factors he was presenting with. Michael was very angry and felt that he wasn't being listened to nor heard.

Katrina took time to reflect how she could encourage Michael to identify his stage of recovery as was known to her from her professional knowledge of the recovery stages of bipolar disorder. Following her reflection, Katrina took time with Michael in a quiet environment to facilitate the discussion that enabled Michael to identify his stage of recovery. Through this discussion a consensus was reached regarding phased opportunities for Michael to spend time at home for brief periods. Michael responded well and was discharged in the care of a community mental health nurse 1 month later.

Morse et al. (2006) also refers to levels of engagement, but in the context of patients who are suffering, and presents an alternative model of communication that is based on two board characteristics:

> (a) whether the nurse is focused on the patient's response (i.e. engaged and, therefore, embodying the sufferer's experience) or focused on self, protecting him/herself from experiencing the patient's suffering, and (b) whether the response is reflexive and spontaneous (first level) or learned (second level) and, therefore, controlled (p. 76).

Morse et al. (2006) describes four positions as (1) *Engaged* (connected response) with behaviours that demonstrate, for example, pity, sympathy and compassion; (2) *Pseudo-engaged* (professional response), with behaviours that demonstrate, for example, sharing self, humour and reassurance; (3) *Anti-engaged* (reflected response), which describes behaviours that demonstrate withdrawing, distancing and labelling; and finally (4) *A-engaged* (detached response), which describes behaviours that are mechanical (rote) and false. Engaged and pseudo-engaged are described as patient focused, whilst *Anti-engaged* and *A-engaged* are described as self-focused. This work is closely aligned to the notion of sympathetic presence, which is discussed in the following section.

*How do I work from person to
   person
Its through the heart and to the
   heart,
Its heart to heart work
Person to person caring.*

The ability to engage and be truly connected with patients is dependent on the nurse's abilities, as reflected in the pre-requisites discussed in Chapter 4. The attributes of expert practice, particularly those that focus on knowing the patient and moral agency, are fundamental to this way of working, as is the clarity of beliefs and values of the nurse and knowing self. As the Framework suggests, however, components within the care environment can have a significant bearing on the nurse's ability to engage with patients in the way that has been described, and further reinforces the need for the nurse to have skills that enables her to manage the care environment to maximise benefits for patients.

Having Sympathetic Presence

The term sympathetic presence has been chosen carefully to describe a way of being with patients that is consistent with person-centredness, but is also achievable in the practice context. Drawing on the original work of McCormack (2001), sympathetic presence is described as 'an engagement that recognises the uniqueness and value of the individual, by appropriately responding to cues that maximise coping resources through the recognition of important agendas in daily life' (p. 270). To have a nurse show, through acceptance of the person, a sympathetic understanding of the patient's losses and present limitations, is to establish a therapeutic relationship, which is directed at gaining an effective outcome from care that is centred on the person's needs and life perspectives. The ability to project a sympathetic presence is therefore dependent on knowing the patient and having insight into their beliefs and values as discussed previously in this chapter.

Presence in the context of person-centred care is something more than simply being physically present. Benner (1984) captures the essence of this when she describes presencing as the art of 'being with' a person without the need to be 'doing to' the person. In an early study by Ford (1990) presence was described as: 'the nurse takes time to listen, she gives her undivided attention to the patient and is able to focus on his needs . . . s/he is authentically present' (p. 160). The following example is drawn from Ford's study and articulates how a nurse made herself present to a patient despite the busy environment.

> *Mr Cook was in the terminal stages of congestive heart failure. He
> had two myocardial infarctions. He was alone, his family were out
> of town. We knew he wasn't doing well. . . . When I touched his
> hand and introduced myself . . . he squeezed my hand and began
> to talk. . . . I sat on his bed, and he reached out and held my hand.
> He talked to me about his life, about his family, and the things he
> wanted to do but wasn't able to. . . . I ignored everything else that
> was going on in the unit at that time: and it was busy. I pulled the
> curtains around one side of the bed because there was some activity
> coming from that side. I just sat and listened as he spoke.*
> *(Ford, 1990: 160)*

There is, however, often a perception that being present is only about sitting with, and talking to, the patient, which can be challenging in the current context where there is often a high turnover of patients and environments are busy. The idea of presence, however, is also interpreted in terms of being attentive or being available. McCance (2003) in her original study describes being attentive as the nurse being present or being visible, often articulated by patients as the nurse 'coming back and forward' or the nurse 'coming in and out'. This also reflects the ability of a nurse to communicate to a patient that they are paying attention even when that can be from a distance, as illustrated from the following story drawn from the Person-Centred Care (PCC) Programme within the Belfast Trust, NI.

Through the day you see them do it, they take a look at you as they walk past you, they are looking after you whether they speak to you or not. You see them walk past, looking and its purely and simply they are judging your situation, whether they do it on purpose or whether its just part of their training. In contrast, there is a few that would walk past here without giving you a once over looking, they don't want to be involved in conversation because they are doing something else but the nurses who have got it they know you are still there.

(McCance et al., 2010)

The perception that person-centred care is mostly about talking to, and spending time with the patient needs to be challenged, particularly in the current health and social care context. We would argue, however, that it is the ability of a nurse to be available to each patient *in that moment*. Every time a patient is approached by a nurse for whatever reason be it to administer medication, to perform a procedure, or to ask a specific question, is an opportunity to be person-centred. There is, however, the potential that being present in this way will uncover issues that need addressed and this can be challenging for a range of reasons. It might be because the nurse doesn't feel confident or lacks the competence to effectively deal with the patient's needs, or indeed it could be a consequence of the environment and the other priorities that are bearing down on the nurse at that time. Furthermore, focusing on tasks can be a defence mechanism, protecting nurses from the emotional labour of nursing work. The following story demonstrates how these issues can manifest in practice.

Jim Smith was forty-five years old when I met him. . . . He was admitted to the cardiopulmonary unit where I was working. The patient had an eight hour history of slurred speech and blurred vision. The symptoms had cleared up prior to his admission and he was now admitted for a diagnostic workup. . . . He was worked up for transitory

(Continued)

ischaemic arterial spasm. Four days later he went home with a negative workup. Two days after that he was readmitted after having a seizure at home. I was on holidays at the time, and by the time I had returned he had a diagnosis of metastic lung cancer. I do not know how he responded to the initial diagnosis – when I returned, I didn't go in to see him for a couple of days. I was really frightened about seeing him because I did not know what to say or do. He made it easy for me, and I did begin working with him again, concentrating on teaching him about chemotherapy and radiotherapy. I felt I was teaching him a lot, but actually he taught me. One day he said to me, "You are doing an OK job Mary, but I can tell that every time you walk in that door you are walking out." He was right. He had developed so much meaning in his illness and life that I was not relating to. This man had really expanded the context of his life into areas where I could have been effective, had I had some understanding.

(Benner & Wrubel, 1989: 16)

It is also important to situate this component of the Framework in the context of the evidence base on empathy. Empathy has been given considerable attention in the nursing literature and is considered highly desirable in nursing practice. The complexity of the concept has been acknowledged and hence several attempts have been made to clarify the terms and its contribution to nursing practice (Burnard, 1988; Gould, 1990; Holden, 1990; Pike, 1990; Morse et al., 1992; Baillie, 1996).

Within the Framework we have chosen to use the term sympathetic as opposed to empathetic and it originates from the essential meaning of these two terms. A simple dictionary definition suggests that empathy is 'the power of projecting one's personality into (and so fully comprehending) the object of contemplation' (Concise Oxford Dictionary, 1976: 338). In contrast, sympathy is defined as 'the quality of being affected by the affection of another, with feelings correspondent in kind, if not in degree; fellow-feeling' (www.dictionary.com). The debate, however, centres around the ability of anyone to be able to fully comprehend another individual's particular experience. Yegdich (1999) from an analysis of this literature base seriously challenges the idea that nurses must first experience all that afflicts their patients, and comments that 'it is analogous to stating that to empathise with a person suffering from a sexually transmitted disease, one must first experience it' (p. 85). Yegdich (1999) argues that sympathy might be more appropriate to nursing, but acknowledges that the nursing literature has given 'less credence to sympathy than to empathy, which has long been given the status of caring' (p. 85). This could be in part attributed to the term sympathy being used to convey pity or feeling sorry for another person, which infers an inward looking position, and can engender thoughts such as: *I am glad I am not there.*

What do you see when you admit me?
New patient? Bed one?
Obs chart and water jug?

What do you see when you look at me?
Uniform of dependence donned in conformity
Night-dressed to legitmise my "patient" rank.

Questions asked of bodily functions,
Your eyes down, recording answers.
Peripheral trivia! Clerked with precision

Please stop.

Look at me – with empathy.
Sense my worry and concern,
See me **the** person that I am.
Respect my hopes, my fears, my prayer
Relate to me – show me you care.

(Poem written by Mrs Liz Henderson,
Director of the Northern Ireland Cancer Network)

The necessity to demonstrate highly developed interpersonal skills is key to being sympathetically present. Furthermore, we would argue that sympathetic presence is the fabric that weaves together other person-centred processes. This idea is also reflected by Titchen (2004) within her Critical Companionship Framework, when she refers to 'graceful care' within the context of relationships. Take for example, providing for a patient's physical needs, which is discussed in detail in the following section as part of providing holistic care. Delivering this aspect of care is dependent on having sympathetic presence, with both elements crucially important for quality outcomes for patients, as demonstrated by the following extract again drawn from the PCC Programme within the Belfast Trust.

When I think of being person-centred I think of a glass bell I have in my cabinet. There are no hidden agendas. Its for the good of all, patients, staff and families. The cut glass reflects the light that comes from reflection. Looking in and on our practice and questioning why and how we do things and ways we can improve enables the glass to shine. And of course the bell rings – when everything comes together in a moment of time!

*I have got a catheter in because that helps another aspect, when you are waiting on a water bottle and you have got like 10 minutes, when you want to use one then you have got to use one, I want one and why do people take them when they are partially full, empty them and don't bring them back. Your problem is heightened by the fact that that water bottle is not there, if it was there you would do your business end of story **but every minute or every second you have to wait to attract the attention of somebody** to get a water bottle and this was doing me no good whatsoever. It was done to help me. When you are trying to find a bottle and you can't breathe, etc., the Dr said the catheter would eliminate the problem that was why it was put in.*

(McCance et al., 2010)

Providing Holistic Care

In the original framework this component focused only on the provision of physical care by a nurse who is professionally competent. We
could argue that this at the heart of nursing work and is reflective
of the essence of nursing as a helping relationship, which provides a
focus for the nurse–patient interaction. The important message in this
component of the Framework is that irrespective of the person-centred
processes discussed above, much of this is often achieved during the
process of delivering technical and physical aspects of care. Indeed it
is argued that registered nurses providing physical care is essential as a
'way in' in order to operationalise other person-centred processes and
to achieve person-centred outcomes (James, 1992; Hallsdorsdottir &
Hamrin, 1997; McCance et al., 1997; McCance, 2003). Furthermore,
there is an emphasis on the importance of provision of competent physical care from the perspective of patients, which has been addressed in
Chapter 4.

In the original framework there was an assumption that the
person-centred processes described would address the psychological
needs of patients, hence the rationale for identifying a theme that
focused solely on providing for physical needs. Consistent feedback,
however, particularly from nurses working in the area of mental
health, encouraged us to explore further the nature of the helping
relationship that characterises nursing. Gamez (2009) describes
the helping relationship as a way of caring for human needs and
concludes:

> The type of interactions in which the nurse participates vary from
> helping patients in activities of daily living to individual group, or
> family therapy. It goes from the individual's home to the hospital
> and to outpatient care. The nurse–patient relationship concentrates
> on needs, the limitations, and the potential of the patient (p. 127).

The identification of patient need is fundamental to several nursing
theories, but the focus is on a range of needs that are more than
just physical or indeed psychological. For example, in the conceptual model derived from mental health nursing developed by Betty
Neuman (1996), her holistic multi-dimensional approach identified
five different variables constituting the client, which she describes
as follows:

> The *physiological variable* refers to bodily structure and function; the
> *psychological variable*, to mental processes and relationships;

the *sociocultural variable*, to social and cultural functions; the *developmental variable* to the developmental processes of life; and the *spiritual variable*, to the influence of spiritual beliefs (p. 225).

Providing holistic care should take account of all these variables and whilst it in not the intention of this book to explore each of these in depth, it is suffice to say that they need to be taken account of when working with patients' beliefs and values in order to meet identified needs.

Psychological support as a nursing intervention has been a focus within the nursing literature. In the original conceptual framework for caring in nursing developed by McCance (2003), there was a component relating to providing psychological care, which reflected activities such as providing information and providing reassurance. The following story demonstrates the close relationship between providing physical care and providing psychological support.

Martha was a 70-year-old lady admitted to a surgical ward with acute abdominal pain and suspected gall stones. Martha had a history of abdominal pain for several months but it was only when she experienced an acute episode and the pain became unbearable that she had to call her GP and was admitted to hospital. When Martha arrived on the ward, the staff worked hard to get her pain under control and by the time the night staff came on duty Martha was well settled. Around 10 p.m. Martha became very distressed and rang for the attention of one of the nurses. A nurse named Ella immediately came to her assistance and asked Martha did she need pain relief. Ella went and got some analgesia to give to Martha and came back a short time later to check if she was feeling any better. Martha was still in pain and by this stage was quietly sobbing. Ella sat down on the bed beside her, took her hand and in a gentle voice asked her what was wrong. Martha began to cry even harder and with Ella's gentle assurance that she was there and listening, she began to talk about her worries about her husband. Fred was Martha's lifelong companion who had been diagnosed with dementia 1 year previously. Martha was devoted to him and took care of his every need and this was the first time they had been apart since he had become unwell, and although her daughter was at home with Fred she was still extremely anxious that he was ok. Ella asked what could she do to ease her worry and Martha said if she could speak to her daughter on the phone she would feel better. Martha was speaking to her daughter less than 5 minutes later, who was able to reassure her that Fred had been well settled all evening and was already in bed asleep. When Martha came of the phone she was so relieved. When Ella called to check on Martha a short time later she was pleased to hear that her pain had eased as well.

A model for professional psychological assessment and support is provided by NICE (2004), but in the context of improving supportive and palliative care for adults with cancer. This model, however, is useful in considering the elements of psychological support more broadly, which are described at four different levels. At level 1, interventions focus on effective information giving, compassion, communication and general psychological support. At level 2, interventions move to psychological techniques such as problem-solving. At level 3, interventions identified include counselling and specific psychological interventions such as anxiety management, and finally at level 4, the focus is on specialist psychological and psychiatric interventions. The intervention used by Ella, the nurse in the above story, reflects an intervention at level 1, where the focus was on picking up important cues through effective communication and acting on these cues in order to provide psychological support. Obviously, the knowledge and skills required to intervene will differ at the various levels, and it relates back to the attributes of the nurse as a fundamental building block in the delivery of effective person-centred care.

Furthermore, there is evidence to suggest that the manner in which physical care is provided can have a significant impact on the patient and this will be discussed in detail in Chapter 7. There is a risk of undertaking physical tasks without paying attention to person-centred processes. In other words, every interaction that involves the provision of physical care is an opportunity to engage with individuals (be they patients, family members or carers) and to work with the principles of person-centredness, as demonstrated from the following extract.

> Here, the good nurses listen to you, I can trust them, you get to know the ones who are good at putting in the cannula, because they listen to you when you point out the good vein. Some junior doctors will not listen, will not chose the vein the patient points out, after failures, I have to say 'get . . . nurse, she/he knows how to do it.
> *(McCance et al., 2010)*

A good example of this, is demonstrated through the randomised control trial conducted by Sloane et al. (2004) who set out to measure the impact of person-centred showering and the towel bath on bathing-associated aggression, agitation and discomfort in nursing home residents with dementia. Person-centred bathing and showering, as defined, appeared to draw on person-centred processes such as working with the patients, beliefs and values and shared decision-making.

Person-centred bathing focused on resident comfort and preferences . . . employed communication techniques appropriate for the resident's level of disease severity and applied problem solving approaches to identify causes and potential solution, and regulated the physical environment to maximise resident comfort. Person-centred showering sought to individualise the experience for the resident by using a wide variety of techniques such as providing choices, covering with towels to maintain resident warmth . . . using bath products recommended by family and staff (p. 1796).

The impact of the interventions above, which were provided by staff who had received person-centred training, measured against the intervention undertaken by staff who received no additional training, produced impressive results on a range of outcome measures. In summary, all measures of agitation and aggression declined significantly in both treatment groups, but not in the control group, as did discomfort scores. Delivering care and paying attention to person-centred processes is at the heart of PCN, but requires nurses who can demonstrate the attributes discussed in Chapter 4.

Accepting the idea that the provision of technical or physical aspects of care are often the way in for operationalising person-centred practice, we must acknowledge that it is not always the nurse who is involved in direct patient care. This is reflective of the move of registered nurses away from direct care provision due to nursing shortages and changes in skill mix. This is further complicated by the increase in the provision of technological care as a result of, for example, the European Working Time Directive and the reduction in junior doctors hours, leading to increased workload for nurses in relation to venepuncture, cannulation and IV administration of medicines and the development of new roles in nursing. This increases the risk of registered nurse providing technical aspects of care and other non-regulated members of the team being left to providing personal care. Furthermore, there is increasing evidence to suggest that skill mix has direct relevance to patient outcomes as a result of the impact of registered nurses. The work of Rafferty et al. (2007) confirmed the relationship between the registered workforce on a range of indicators such as mortality, job satisfaction, burnout and quality of care. They concluded that hospitals with more favourable staffing levels had consistently better outcomes than those hospitals with less favourable staffing. The impact of person-centred practice, however, and the identification of indicators that reflect the contribution of nurses to patient outcomes that reflect their care experience are less evident in the nursing literature (National Nursing Research Unit, 2008).

Meanwhile in St Josephs Unit

In the unit of St Josephs you won't hear too much noise
Some of us are silent an odd one sits and sighs

But look behind the faces and put away the chart
I'm sure my pulse is normal but try to read my heart.

In my years before St Josephs I had some golden hours
And I walked with my true love among leafy bowers
And if my eyes look vacant and sometimes I don't hear
I may be gone to shelter from the rain that fills my tears.

There was a time believe me when friends were near and dear
And I drank the cup of kindness and laughed without a fear
So when you think I'm hungry and I push away the food
I am struggling with my demons and don't mean to be rude.

And, staff, I do take notice when you greet me with a smile
And I really mean to thank you when you go the extra mile
But sometimes I am angry though I know it doesn't help
And when you lose your patience I can only blame myself.

In the unit of St Josephs there are some who dare to hope
And some whose hopes are fading feel like giving up the ghost
But life is very precious though the deal you got is raw
There's no room for self-pity with your back against the wall.

So please listen to my story and try to make the time
You might just learn a lesson and be a bit more wise
I will try hard to respond and not be such a pain
With a little understanding we both can stand to gain.

In the unit of St Josephs life may seem very bleak
But life is still worth living for the sad and for the weak
And one thing is for certain as you go about your chore
The day is so much brighter when you look into my soul.

(Anonymous)

Summary of Key Points

The person-centred processes presented in the PCN Framework and discussed in this chapter, reflect key elements of the interactions between patients and nurses. Gaining an understanding of an individual's value base and being able to work with their beliefs and values to facilitate shared decision-making is essential to PCN. Furthermore, there is an emphasis on holistic care and the breath of potential nursing interventions required to meet identified need. Being engaged in a way that enables sympathetic presence is the vehicle for the delivering person-centred processes. Whilst it is acknowledged that the demands of everyday nursing practice can often work against the person-centred approach described in this chapter, it is also recognised that there is potential for much attitudinal and behavioural change that could enable this philosophy to be achieved. This further reinforces relationships in the model between the attributes of the nurse and the care environment, which need to be conducive for the delivery of person-centred processes.

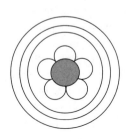

Chapter 7

Person-Centred Nursing Outcomes and their Evaluation

Introduction

Outcomes are the results expected from effective PCN. The literature on PCN is weak in terms of methods for evaluating outcomes, with little clarity about outcome focus, methodologies or methods. We have identified three themes for outcome measurement. Outcomes in these themes can be demonstrated from the perspectives of both staff and patients/families. In this chapter, we will explore these three themes from the perspectives of challenges, approaches and tools (Figure 7.1).

The chapter will begin with an overview of outcome evaluation in nursing with a particular focus on how caring outcomes are reflected in the literature. The challenges associated with determining outcomes from PCN will then be discussed. A framework for evaluating outcomes from PCN will be proposed that takes account of the evaluation of processes and outcomes arising. Finally, the chapter will propose a variety of methods that can be used to evaluate PCN outcomes.

Outcome Evaluation in Nursing

Measuring the effectiveness of nursing is problematic. There is a large and diverse literature that attempts to determine both the key indicators for outcome measurement and methodological approaches. The nursing literature also highlights the challenges associated with evaluating the effectiveness of nursing due to the

Figure 7.1 Person-centred outcomes themes.

- feeling involved in care,
- having a feeling of well-being,
- the existence of a therapeutic environment, described as one in which:
  - decision-making is shared,
  - staff relationships are collaborative,
  - leadership is transformational,
  - innovative practices are supported.

diversity of perspectives and frameworks that underpin the practice of nursing. The challenges associated with what has been referred to as 'the invisibility' of nursing is also a significant issue in the evaluation of nursing outcomes. The invisibility argument refers to the nature of nursing practice itself. Unlike other health care professionals, many nursing practices cannot be delineated as specific interventions where there is a clear input matched to an outcome – for example, a physiotherapist can evaluate their input to a patient's improvement following a fractured neck of femur repair in terms of the number and types of specific treatments (interventions) offered and the rate of improvement determined by the objective measurement of movement. Much of the work of other health care professionals (e.g. physiotherapists) is treatment or intervention specific and thus the outcome from these interventions has greater potential for outcome evaluation.

Nursing on the other hand, whilst engaging in specific treatment interventions, often does so as a part of an ongoing and continuous engagement with patients/service users and so aspects of practice associated with providing a specific intervention (such as administration of intravenous therapies, treatment of a pressure sore or assisting with nutrition) are 'hidden' and not visible or open to objective measurement. In a discussion paper, McQueen (2000) highlights the incongruity that exists between models of care that emphasise the importance of therapeutic relationships between patients, families and care staff, whilst at the same time little emphasis is placed on these activities in the measurement of nursing outcomes. McQueen (2000) argues that if nurses are required in this way, then the interpersonal and emotional nature of the work needs to be recognised in clinical practice, education and research and be included in the way that nursing effectiveness is measured and evaluated.

Staff nurse Orla Dempsey works in an acute medical ward where she is a primary nurse to six patients, each of whom have varied care needs. Orla is on duty with a care assistant (nurses aide). At the beginning of the shift, Orla undertakes an assessment of the care needs of the patients she is working with in order to determine how best to plan her work and that of the care assistant (nurses aide) for the shift. Some patients have very specific 'technical' care inputs that Orla is able to clearly identify and to which she can allocate a specific period of time. The rest of their care needs can largely be met by the care assistant (nurses aide) with Orla's supervision. The remainder of the patients have more complex care needs that include technical interventions. Orla prioritises these patients as those she will dedicate most time to and in planning their care includes the technical interventions. She builds these into the overall plan of care.

During the shift, the care assistant approaches Orla and lets her know that Shaun, one of the patients whom she has been allocated, needs his intravenous nutrition replaced as the previous one is complete. Orla views this as a 'straightforward' and 'uncomplicated' task to do. However, whilst chatting with Shaun during the procedure she discovers that Shaun is deeply concerned about how he will resume his sexual relationship with his partner. Orla spends an hour talking this through with Shaun, discussing options with him and identifying sources of support, as well as attending to other aspects of his physical care needs.

Later in the day, whilst completing the workload allocation record for a 'nursing workload audit', Orla documents her work with Shaun under two headings – 'specific treatment' and 'patient support'. However, she feels deeply dissatisfied with this as she knows that during that time she also provided comfort, engagement, empathy and personal care but it is not possible to show these in the audit record.

Some authors are critical of the 'invisibility' and 'hidden' arguments in health care practice and suggest that these arguments are more reflective of the need to understand 'complexity' in many health care practices (Plsek & Greenhalgh, 2001; Cutliffe & Wieck, 2008). The complexity of nursing is a key consideration and helps to make sense of why nursing effectiveness cannot be judged on 'output' alone, but that there need to be frameworks developed that evaluate outputs/outcomes in relation to inputs (Spilsbury & Meyer, 2000; Meyer & Sturdy, 2004). Internationally, much work has been undertaken on determining outcome indicators for nursing by organisations such as The International Council of Nursing (ICN) (development of nursing-sensitive outcome indicators http://www.icn.ch/matters_indicators .htm) and the National Database of Nursing Quality Indicators in the United States (Montalvo, 2007). In addition, research into the 'expertise of nursing' has begun to identify the complexity of nursing work and the importance of evaluating the effectiveness of this work beyond simple input/output models (Hardy et al., 2009).

A recent review of aspects of nursing linked to patient outcome from the UK 'National Nursing Research Unit' (Policy + 2008) highlighted the complexity of measuring outcomes in patient care. The authors highlighted 'failure to rescue' and health care-associated infection as nurse-sensitive outcomes, but falls and pressure sores were less sensitive. They also highlight that positive contributions of nursing to outcomes such as well-being or recovery are less well addressed in nursing outcome frameworks. However, Maben and Griffiths (2008) highlight those aspects of care that patients most value, including:

- A holistic approach to physical, mental and emotional needs, patient-centred and continuous care.
- Efficiency and effectiveness combined with humanity and compassion.
- Professional, high-quality evidence-based practice.
- Safe, effective and prompt nursing interventions.

- Patient empowerment, support and advocacy.
- Seamless care through effective teamwork with other professions.

These aspects of patient care feature less strongly in nursing outcomes frameworks but yet are consistent with the principles and values underpinning PCN.

Outcome Evaluation in Person-Centred Nursing

The evaluation of nursing specific outcomes arising from the adoption of a person-centred approach to practice is underdeveloped and there are few reports of published person-centred outcome evaluation in the literature. Whilst the principles and values of person-centred care/nursing are enshrined in much contemporary nursing and health care policy and strategy, the empirical evidence available to support it as an operational framework for nursing and health care delivery is as yet unconvincing. Descriptive accounts of PCN leave little doubt that it does impact on patient's experience of care services and nurses experiences of caring. However, there is a need to develop creative strategies for evaluating the complex processes that underpin person-centredness in practice.

Research in areas of vulnerable people such as older people and people with intellectual disabilities has shown it to be effective in promoting patient choice, improving the experience of being cared for and patient involvement in care (Parley, 2001; Dewing, 2002; Clarke et al., 2003). Despite this, the evidence to support its impact on nursing is sparse. Attempts have been made to evaluate the impact of PCN in specific aspects of care, for example, the impact of person-centred showering (bathing) on bathing-associated aggression, agitation and discomfort in nursing home residents with dementia (Sloane et al., 2004; Hoeffer et al., 2006), the impact of multisensory environments on older people with dementia (Hope & Waterman, 2004), the evaluation of the development of 'relationship skills' between nurses aides and patients (Medvene et al., 2006) and exploration of how preceptors interpret, operationalise, document and teach person-centred care with students in a surgical setting (McCarthy, 2006). Other studies have evaluated person-centred planning with people with intellectual disabilities (Robertson et al., 2007), the experience of woman-centred care (Pope et al., 2001) and a number of studies that have evaluated the impact of person-centred care on people with dementia from a variety of perspectives (Dewing, 2008c).

Person-centred nursing, as a model, reports the advancement of traits such as adequate staffing levels, decentralised structures, professional practice models of delivery and professional development issues (Binnie & Titchen, 1999) as a result of systems changes adopted to facilitate its implementation.

The work of Binnie and Titchen (1999) remains one of the few studies that systematically analysed development of a person-centred culture in an acute care setting[1]. Evidence from Binnie and Titchen's research suggested that adopting this approach to nursing provides more holistic care. In addition, it may increase patient satisfaction with the level of care, reduce anxiety levels among nurses in the long term and promote team working among staff. Binnie and Titchen, however, did not test these assertions and were therefore unable to provide evidence of the suggested relationships.

Existing evidence is consistent with the view that being person-centred requires the formation of therapeutic relationships between professionals, patients and others significant to them in their lives and that these relationships are built on mutual trust, understanding and a sharing of collective knowledge (Binnie & Titchen, 1999; Dewing, 2004; McCormack, 2004; Nolan et al., 2004). Binnie and Titchen (1999) tried to make explicit what is a nurse–patient therapeutic relationship. They highlighted the importance of the nurse avoiding the making of assumptions about patients, being ready to listen and to watch with an open mind. The emphasis on skills is essential, both in terms of practical skill and trained presence. This approach requires intelligence, creativity and attention to detail, and transforms the focus of bedside care:

> in skilled hands, the opportunities presented by everyday bedside caring become the medium through which a patient's experience of illness can be transformed.

> (Binnie & Titchen, 1999: 18)

We have already suggested that life plans of the individual and enabling and disabling aspects of the context of the care environment are important considerations in PCN. The context of care was seen as having the greatest potential to help or hinder the facilitation of PCN.

In modern health care, the fundamental moral situation of nurses is that whilst they are expected to engage in autonomous decision-making, they are often deprived of the freedom to exercise moral authority. To exercise their freedom requires nurses to ask questions of their traditional methods of nursing, and having the belief that they can and should change the context of care. The context of care extends beyond autonomy to practice, and can be found, with equal significance, in other organisational factors such as systems of decision-making, staff relationships, organisational systems, power differentials and the potential of the organisation to tolerate innovate practices and risk-taking (McCormack et al., 2002).

Hale (1986), using a simple version of PCN, found increased levels of job satisfaction and morale among the staff; nursing stress levels also decreased. Johns (1994) and Ellis (1999) reported similar results. Ellis added that PCN 'enhanced oneself, ones practice, professional education and the organisation as a whole' (p. 300), thus highlighting the importance of the evaluation of PCN extending beyond direct patient outcomes, and including staff and organisational outcomes.

Complementary evidence from research such as magnet hospitals and models of nursing practice shows that changing an organisations' culture has an impact on the issues concerning nurses working life

(Hayes et al., 2006; Manojlovich & Laschinger, 2007; Gunnarsdóttir et al., 2009). The bulk of this evidence draws a causal link between organisational culture change and working environment factors such as retention of staff, job satisfaction and job stress. Yet, Newman et al. (2001) found that, in the United Kingdom, there has been no unified or cohesive approach to workplace planning. The researchers state that there is a governmental acknowledgement of and commitment to the importance of the organisational culture in promoting nurse retention, job satisfaction and reduced stress, yet this commitment has not manifested itself into a single method of implementation (Newman et al., 2001). The Institute of Medicine in the United States reiterated the importance of organisational culture as an aspect of improving nurses' working environment and proposed guidelines for hospitals based on research conducted into 'magnet hospitals' where it identified a number of traits such as professional autonomy and practice control as key in keeping nurses working. The report authors concluded that:

> Quality problems (nurse retention and patient satisfaction levels) occur typically not because of a failure of goodwill, knowledge, effort, or resources devoted to health care, but because of fundamental shortcomings in the way care is organised.

> (2001: 25).

Person-centred nursing involves the reorganisation of the context of care to promote continuity of care, amongst other things (McCormack, 2003, 2004). The context of care offers the greatest source of facilitation (or hindrance) to the development of a person-centred ethos in the nurse's workplace (Manley, 2001; McCormack, 2004). Whilst overall, there is a lack of outcome evaluation in PCN, the potential benefits of PCN to patients is more often documented (Parley, 2001; Dewing, 2002; Clarke et al., 2003), with the benefits to nurses not so clearly articulated. The research that exists reports the advancement of traits such as adequate staffing levels, decentralised structures, professional practice models of delivery and professional development issues (Binnie & Titchen, 1999) and with these changes reduced stress levels, increased job satisfaction and nurse retention. Research into organisational culture supports the link between decentralised structures, autonomy and nurse satisfaction and retention (Hayes et al., 2006; O'Brien-Pallas, 2008).

In summary, whilst the values and principles of PCN are increasingly espoused in policy and strategy, its evaluation and particularly outcome evaluation is poorly developed. Whilst debates persist about the meaning of underpinning concepts, the appropriateness of models and their implementation, approaches to outcome evaluation receive less attention. Some of this lack of attention is due to the limitations of existing methodologies to capture the complexity of PCN in its entirety and thus it is easier to evaluate sub-elements. In addition, few instruments measure constructs such as 'patient involvement in care' and there are few conceptual frameworks of patient satisfaction that explicitly include patient involvement. Previous research and development work focusing on caring in nursing highlights that perceptions differed between patients and nurses, which is discussed in Chapters 3 and 4. Such challenges highlight the need for evaluation frameworks that capture the complexity of the interrelationships of the elements of PCN if it is to be embedded in practice. It is this challenge that we will next address.

A Framework for Outcome Evaluation

In the PCN Framework presented in this book, we have identified four outcomes that would be achieved from the development of a PCN culture:

1. satisfaction with care
2. involvement with care
3. feeling of well-being
4. creating a therapeutic culture

Satisfaction with care is a well-established outcome measure in nursing and health care. However, it is also one of the most challenging outcomes to evaluate. The challenges in evaluating satisfaction with care are many – an inability to determine a universally accepted definition of 'satisfaction', the multiple meanings attached to the term that are often highly individualised and idiosyncratic and the lack of comprehensive measurement tools to capture the multidimensionality of the term (Staniszewska & Ahmed, 1999; Edwards & Staniszewska, 2000; Edwards et al., 2004; Entwistle et al., 2004; Entwistle & Watt, 2006). The evaluation of patient satisfaction is often reduced to the level of organisational audit where annual patient satisfaction surveys are a key approach to determining the effectiveness of an organisation. However, such surveys lack depth, fail to capture individual perspectives of satisfaction and lack conceptual rigour (Edwards et al., 2004). From the perspective of PCN, evaluating satisfaction cannot rely on organisational-wide surveys, instead the effectiveness of the care processes and the care context (environment of care) to support these should be central.

Feeling involved in care is a key part of contemporary health care strategy and policy and there is an explicit expectation that patients will be active participants in their own care. Examples such as 'the expert patient initiative' are predicated on the assumption that people will be active participants in their care and work in partnership with health care professionals. Thus evaluating the extent to which people feel involved in their care would seem to be a key focus of person-centred outcome evaluation. In addition from a staff perspective, being involved in the decision-making process is a key focus of many models of care that aim to ensure that care decisions are made by nurses working directly with patients and is a key indicator in developments such as the magnet hospitals.

Having a feeling of well-being underpins the aims of many caring theories, rehabilitation models and care practices. McCance (2003) clearly articulated how positive care experiences engendered feelings of well-being among patients and is indicative of the patient being valued. Similarly, nurses need to feel valued for their work and thus is also considered a key aspect of outcome evaluation in PCN.

Creating a therapeutic culture has been demonstrated to a key factor in the delivery of PCN and the extent to which the environment supports and maintains person-centred principles has been shown to be critical to PCN.

In a study aimed at 'shifting the culture of practice' in an acute care setting through the introduction of an integrated work-based learning/research/practice development framework (known as the REACH Framework), Boomer et al. (2006) created a conceptual framework for evaluating relationships between structure, process and outcome elements of the REACH programme of work (Figure 7.2).

The ultimate aim of the REACH programme is that of creating a person-centred culture. Evidence from research and development underpinning the REACH Framework indicates four types

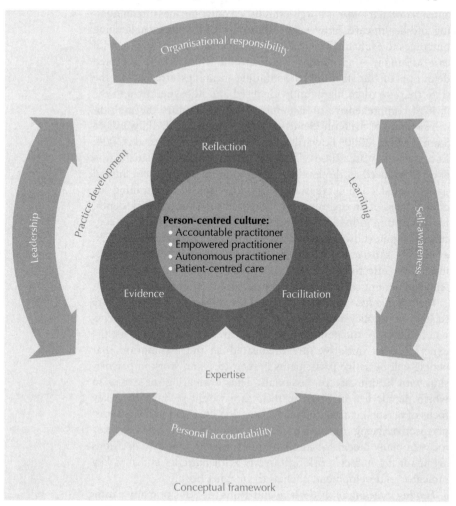

Figure 7.2 The REACH conceptual framework.

of outcomes – accountable practitioners, empowered practitioners, autonomous practitioners and the delivery of patient-centred care. In order to achieve these outcomes, three layers of activity are needed:

1. learning mechanisms
2. practice domains
3. individual and organisational responsibility

The learning mechanisms (reflection, facilitation and evidence) are key to enabling learning to happen. Drawing on a variety of evidence sources and reflecting on the processes and outcomes of these different types of evidence through facilitated processes has been shown to contribute to the creation of cultures of effectiveness (Manley, 2000b). In the REACH Framework, assessment of nursing expertise and progress with developing expertise is undertaken using an attributes framework. The attributes framework has 28 attributes of nursing expertise. These are divided into three practice domains or groupings: learning, expertise and practice development. The attributes are not skills-based competencies but instead are seen as the qualities and traits of nursing expertise. They are generic across all nursing roles, levels or bands and are therefore transferable across an organisation. The practice domains form the foci for the development of practice. Finally, individual and organisational responsibility is needed if learning is to occur and practice is to change. Consistent with other international evidence, such as that of the magnet hospitals movement, the research of Boomer et al. (2006) identified organisational responsibility, leadership, personal accountability and self-awareness as being key to developing and sustaining a person-centred culture. The commitment from the organisation is demonstrated in the form of resources, support, valuing of staff, receptiveness to change and a commitment to transformational leadership. This leadership is required at multiple levels and is usually epitomised in the vision statement of the organisation. Effective leadership requires a high level of self-awareness and personal accountability and it is argued that within this framework this can be achieved by the development activities (practice domains) and the culture of challenge with support (Wilson et al., 2006) created by operationalising the learning mechanisms (reflection, evidence and facilitation).

Through combining the research of McCormack and McCance (2006) and Boomer et al. (2006) (Figure 7.3), an outcomes framework can be developed that captures the key dimensions of PCN, set within a person-centred culture.

A realistic approach to evaluating outcomes

Figure 7.3 sets out the five constructs that can be evaluated in the context of PCN:

1. satisfaction with care
2. involvement with care
3. nursing well-being

4. the existence of a therapeutic culture
5. enablers of person-centred cultures

A realistic evaluation approach provides a useful way of framing these constructs into a holistic evaluation framework. Pawson and Tilley (1997) contend that realistic evaluation offers researchers the opportunity to look at evaluation from a real-world perspective. Realistic evaluation was developed with the aim of trying to overcome some of the difficulties encountered with measurement and the effects of causation within complex social systems. Pawson and Tilley (1997) argue that evaluations of social programmes take place in environments that are rapidly changing and in which the setting is just as important as the intervention being evaluated. Therefore, it is important to go beyond the study of the usual cause and effect relationships that are emphasised in more traditional approaches to evaluation. Therefore rather than asking if the intervention works, or comparing one intervention to another, realistic evaluation sets out to answer 'what is it about a programme that works (the mechanisms of change), why it works, for whom it works, and in what circumstances it works'. Pawson and Tilley (1997) developed the following formula to represent this: Context (C) + Mechanism (M) = Outcome (O).

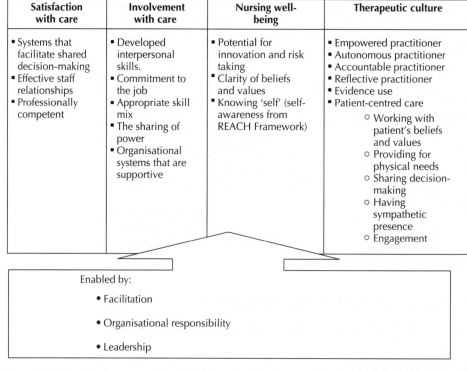

Satisfaction with care	Involvement with care	Nursing well-being	Therapeutic culture

▪ Systems that facilitate shared decision-making
▪ Effective staff relationships
▪ Professionally competent
	▪ Developed interpersonal skills.
	▪ Commitment to the job
	▪ Appropriate skill mix
	▪ The sharing of power
	▪ Organisational systems that are supportive
		▪ Potential for innovation and risk taking
		▪ Clarity of beliefs and values
		▪ Knowing 'self' (self-awareness from REACH Framework)
			▪ Empowered practitioner
			▪ Autonomous practitioner
			▪ Accountable practitioner
			▪ Reflective practitioner
			▪ Evidence use
			▪ Patient-centred care
			  ○ Working with patient's beliefs and values
			  ○ Providing for physical needs
			  ○ Sharing decision-making
			  ○ Having sympathetic presence
			  ○ Engagement

Enabled by:

• Facilitation

• Organisational responsibility

• Leadership

Figure 7.3 Mapping of outcomes related foci from the PCN Framework (McCormack & McCance, 2006) and the REACH Framework (Boomer et al., 2006).

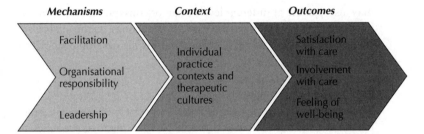

Figure 7.4 Mechanisms, context, outcomes evaluation framework.

This means a programme (such as the development of PCN) includes all the players (e.g. teams, patients, families), the venue (the setting in which person-centredness is being developed) with its past and its history. Mechanisms for change are formed by identifying the capacities (e.g. potential for change), resources (e.g. people), constraints and choices (e.g. identified need for change) facing key stakeholders. The relationship between the mechanism and the outcome is dependent upon the context or location and social norms, that is where it takes place and how the rules of that place influence the mechanism and outcome. Therefore, the evaluator is looking to see what implications the existing context has on the success or failure of the intervention, what the context–mechanism–outcome configuration is and how this can influence the future development of interventions.

Realistic evaluation takes into account both the process and context of change. This results in exploration not only of outcomes but also of conditions that were present to enable those outcomes to occur – something that has been argued for earlier in the context of determining outcomes from nursing interventions. Tolson (1999) and Redfern et al. (2003) suggest that realistic evaluation placed within research and practice presents nurses with a tactical resolution to evaluating innovative nursing practice and offers an explanatory dimension to evaluation.

Therefore, considering the five constructs that can be used to evaluate PCN, the adoption of a realistic evaluation approach lends itself to developing evaluation frameworks that take account of the processes used to develop person-centredness (mechanisms), the settings within which the developments take place (context) and the resulting outcomes (Figure 7.4).

Methods for operationalising the outcome evaluation framework

Mechanisms

In our framework, the mechanisms for enabling PCN (facilitation, organisational responsibility and leadership) operate at an organisational level, that these are mechanisms that need to be in place/ enabled to be in place in order for an organisation to demonstrate corporate responsibility for person-centredness. However, mechanisms may also operate at different levels of an organisation and this will be illustrated further when we discuss 'context' issues, as the analysis of the practice context will trigger mechanisms for development at this level also.

Facilitation

The term 'facilitation' is used to describe a variety of activities, ranging from teaching activities through to humanistic approaches to enabling others. At its simplest, facilitation means *'a technique by which one person makes things easier for others'* (Kitson et al., 1998).

More recently, Shaw et al. (2008) have defined facilitation as being about:

> a helping relationship, essentially one of enabling others and consequently self, through transitions to achieve growth/development and ultimately self-actualisation.
>
> (Shaw et al., 2008)

Harvey et al. (2002) state that the concept of facilitation appears to have emerged from the fields of counselling and student-centred learning, influenced in particular by the work of Carl Rogers (1969). In Roger's work and subsequent developments (e.g. by Heron, 1989), facilitation refers to a process of enabling individuals and groups to understand the processes they have to go through to change aspects of their behaviour or attitudes to themselves, their work or other individuals.

Shaw et al. (2008) have drawn on a broad range of ideas both from co-learners and from the literature in facilitation and humanistic caring (Carl Rogers, 1969; Mayeroff, 1971; Swanson, 1991, 1993; Dewey, 2004), all of which is underpinned by a particular view of persons and personhood. Enabling as caring recognises and accommodates the four different modes of being in the world according to certain philosophies, in that it focuses on helping relationships, the importance of the person and transitions (which requires addressing issues of context) and growth/development.

Much of the work that a facilitator will do is with groups as well as with individuals on a 1:1 basis. The work of John Heron can be very useful here. Heron (1989) describes a facilitator as a person who has the role of helping participants to learn in an experiential group. He believes that an effective facilitator who wants to provide conditions for the development of autonomous learning moves between three political modes: making decisions for learners (hierarchy), making decisions with learners (co-operation) and delegating decisions to learners (autonomy).

Heron emphasises the facilitator's role in addressing issues of feelings within the group, confronting resistance and giving meaning to group discussions; however, he also acknowledges their role in planning and structuring the tasks (from Harvey et al., 2002). This introductory overview of the different ways in which the term 'facilitation' is conceptualised raises issues about how our knowledge influences the types of facilitation we can offer and also how facilitation approaches need to be targeted appropriately in order to help individuals and groups access different knowledge sources.

The quality of the facilitation relationship can be evaluated through a range of methods, including:

- Structured individual and group feedback on the process used by the facilitator to enable effective individual and group engagement.
- Focus group discussions with participants on the effectiveness of (for example) group processes, how the individual addressed individual needs and concerns and the experience of achieving particular tasks.
- Reflective reviews by individual participants and the facilitator.
- Mapping of 'key learning' achieved by individual participants as the work progresses.
- 360-degree feedback (Garbett et al., 2007) of facilitator effectiveness. 360-degree feedback has been defined as 'The systematic collection and feedback of performance data on an individual or group derived from a number of stakeholders in their performance' (Ward, 1997: 4).
- Mapping of 'action points' agreed and implemented by participants and evaluation of their perceptions of the outcomes arising from the implementation of the action points.

Organisational responsibility

The primary responsibility of organisations is that of providing the conditions for clinical teams to continuously evaluate their effectiveness in developing person-centred cultures. Attributes of organisations that act as mechanisms for supporting the development of PCN include:

- *Shared governance approach to nursing management*: In this culture, everybody is seen as a leader of something and accountability and autonomy is actively promoted among staff at every level to lead.
- *Continuous quality improvement*: The organisation needs to foster a culture that views quality as being everybody's business.
- *The existence of an explicit person-centred philosophy*: This philosophy is reflected in the way practice is organised, how staff are employed and the support mechanisms in place for staff, patients, families and communities.
- *Availability of resources for evidence-informed practice*: The organisation fosters a culture of shared evidence-informed decision-making between practitioner, patient and others significant to them, through its governance structures and processes. Evidence-informed practice is the process of shared decision-making based on *research evidence, the patient's experiences and preferences, clinical expertise or know-how* and *other available robust sources of information* (Rycroft Malone et al., 2003). The blending of

these different types of evidence in the decision-making process may be influenced by factors in the practice context such as available resources, practice cultures and norms, leadership styles and data management. The outcome of the decision-making process should be person-centred, evidence-informed care.

- *A reflective approach to feedback* from patients is welcomed and valued at a clinical practice level and patients are encouraged and enabled to reflect on their health and social care experience. Such feedback from patients is welcomed and actively used to continuously develop practice. In working with such feedback and quality improvement, practitioners are active participants in evidence generation and utilisation. Nursing leaders create a culture where evidence utilisation and generation is an explicit part of practice.
- *Clinical leadership and clinical expertise is valued in management frameworks*: The central remit of the nurse leader is that of practice developer. He/she does this by role-modelling expertise in practice, creating a culture where person-centredness can flourish, enabling critical inquiry to happen through a variety of approaches (including supervision, supported reflection, staff meetings), actively seeking feedback from service users, working in partnership with staff members and utilising internal and external policy developments as opportunities for further development and improvement.
- *Systematic and continuous evaluation*: There is a systematic approach to the evaluation of practice achievements through clinical audit, patient stories and organisational review. Activity reports are made accessible to the public and achievements, no matter how small, are celebrated.

In such a culture, learning is an explicit component of practice. To facilitate the process of learning from experience, there needs to be organisational support for the principles and values underpinning practitioner research (McCormack, 2009), combined with an infrastructure that systematically assists nurses to reflect on practice experience, critically review the elements of that practice, actively engage in developing/experimenting with practice and synthesising the learning gained from the process.

For this culture to be created, criticism needs not to be suppressed (as a threat or an act of blaming) but is instead welcomed as a part of a continuous learning process. Evaluation of practice in this culture does not rely solely on managerial-driven agendas of efficiency and effectiveness in order to demonstrate corporate accountability. Instead, evaluation is seen as 'self-evaluation' utilising a variety of approaches including feedback from colleagues, feedback from service users and feedback from service leaders in a continuous cycle of improvement. For such evaluations to be genuinely of value, they must lead to action – actions that are instigated and owned by practitioners and supported by service leaders at every level. Responsibility for such actions lies with practice leaders, as they are set within the boundaries of broad corporate goals of the organisation. Thus the organisation demonstrates trust among practitioners to exercise their autonomy. Leadership is central to this culture and everybody is seen as a leader of something (transformational leadership). Knowledge generated externally (e.g. from academic communities, professional bodies and statutory organisations) is welcomed in that it helps to place local developments in a strategic context. Creating such a culture does not (in the first instance) require the establishment of 'new' structures. However, it does require:

- A commitment to clarifying and making explicit values underpinning practice.
- Embracing transformational leadership.
- Being systematic and rigorous in operationalising person-centredness.
- Commitment to making person-centredness happen.
- Role clarity among leaders and 'enablers' of a person-centred culture.

Leadership

The importance of nursing leadership is well documented. Since the evolution of nursing through organisational models and frameworks that promote individual autonomy, decentralised decision-making and devolution of control over practice to the 'point of care delivery', the need for nurses to engage in leadership styles that are facilitative rather than hierarchical and controlling has increased (Porter-O'Grady, 2003). The most widely recognised model of leadership in nursing and the one most often cited in contemporary nursing is that of transformational leadership (Kouzes & Posner, 2007).

According to Kouzes and Posner (2007) people follow leaders who inspire them, show passion and vision and who inject enthusiasm and passion for their work. Transformational leadership is characterised by having shared values and vision, adopting a facilitative and enabling approach, role-modelling of expertise, promotion of autonomy, empowerment, reflective feedback and celebration of achievements. Transformational leaders focus on building strong and effective teams and in nursing has been shown to be effective in developing evidence-informed and person-centred practice cultures (Cunningham & Kitson, 2000a,b; Large et al., 2005; Shaw, 2005). Through the study of leaders, Kouzes and Posner have identified the most favoured characteristics of leaders (in order of preference):

- honest
- forward-looking
- competent
- inspiring
- intelligent
- fair-minded
- broad-minded

- supportive
- straightforward
- dependable
- cooperative
- determined
- imaginative
- ambitious
- courageous
- caring
- mature
- loyal
- self-controlled
- independent

A leader who has a well-developed 'vision' is essential to transformational leadership. The vision must be developed by the leader and then processes put in place to constantly sell the vision to others (followers). Whilst the importance of a vision for practice or a service is essential, we would argue that the idea of the leader developing the vision and then 'selling' it is limited. Evidence suggests that the need for teams to own the vision is essential to transformation and thus approaches to developing a 'shared vision' between leaders and teams should be adopted (Cunningham & Kitson, 2000a,b; refs). We would suggest that leaders should work with teams to develop a shared vision for person-centredness. Developing change strategies, planning actions and engaging in collaborative relationships towards implementation of changes is more likely to be shared among teams if there is initial ownership of the vision.

To demonstrate transformational leadership in action, Kouzes and Posner outline five core practices of transformational leaders and these are presented here as they are consistent with the values underpinning PCN and thus offer a framework for reflecting on and evaluating the effectiveness of leadership practices for PCN:

- *Inspire a shared vision:* If leaders are to be followed, then people need to understand where it is they are going! A leader needs to have a vision for PCN and how it would ideally 'look' and 'be lived' in practice. The vision needs to be articulated to others and in the inspiration of others, the leader generates a culture of dialogue where the vision becomes 'infectious' and owned by all.
- *Model the way:* What leaders *do* is far more important than what they *say*. They set the example for expected behaviours through their daily actions that demonstrate their commitment to stated values and beliefs. In order to do this effectively of course, an organisation needs to have explicit shared values about person-centred practice and how it is intended to be realised in the organisation.
- *Challenge the process:* A transformational leader doesn't accept the 'status quo'. Leaders continuously search for opportunities to

innovate, grow and develop, that is generate a culture of continuous quality improvement. Because of their commitment to a shared vision, leaders continuously strive for 'better practice' whilst always acknowledging and celebrating achievements along the way. Not all new ideas come from the leader, instead individuals in teams also generate new ideas and the role of the leader is to support the new idea and be willing to challenge the system in order to get the new ideas adopted and converted into everyday practice.

- *Enable others to act:* The leader is a facilitator of change, development and innovation. A systematic approach is adopted to the planning of developments and in the support of participants along the way. Leaders are enablers and as such they facilitate critical dialogue, contestation and debate as it is through these processes that active problem-solving and creative solutions are realised.
- *Encourage the heart:* A leader needs to set clear standards so that people know what is expected of them. Through generating a culture that values individual contributions to continuous improvement and showing that they 'expect the best', leaders generate a 'self-fulfilling prophecy'. Leaders need to be attentive to individual journeys as the change progresses and recognises the contribution of individuals and teams. Successes need to be celebrated as a team and the story of the development journey is told in recognition of success.

The 'Leadership Practices Inventory' was developed by Kouzes and Posner and it evaluates these five dimensions of leadership. The instrument has well-established validity and reliability and has been widely used in a number of studies (Kouzes & Posner, 2002, 2003; McNeese-Smith, 1993, 1995; Cunningham & Kitson, 2000a,b; Large et al., 2005) and continues to be the instrument of choice in many studies of leadership in nursing. The use of such an instrument can also be complemented with qualitative evaluation such as focus groups, individual interviews, reflective conversations and values clarification.

Points to Ponder

Consider your own organisational context and the 'enablers' of person-centredness identified here. Consider the following questions:

1. How do these enablers reflect your own organisation?
2. Does your organisation have an explicit focus on developing person-centred cultures?
3. What could you do to initiate discussion or build support for developing 'organisational responsibility' for person-centredness?

Context

Evaluating the context of practice and the existence of person-centred values and behaviours is an essential step in developing PCN. Knowing what aspects of the practice context are consistent with the values underpinning PCN, what behaviours are inconsistent with those values and thus identifying what aspects of practice need to change are critical to the identification of the most appropriate development 'mechanisms'.

Two approaches to evaluating practice context are offered – The 'Context Assessment Index' (CAI) (McCormack et al., 2009) and the 'Workplace Culture Critical Analysis Tool' (WCCAT) (McCormack et al., 2009a).

The *CAI* (McCormack et al., 2009b) was developed as an instrument for identifying the aspects of practice context that enable person-centred practices and those that need to be further developed. The aim of the CAI is to enable health care professionals to assess the context within which care is provided in clinical areas. It can be completed by one person such as a specialist or ward leader, or the tool can be completed by each member of the team. It is recommended that one person coordinates the process.

Context is defined as the setting or environment where people receive health care services. Three elements have been identified that form the context to ensure there is person-centred practice (McCormack et al., 2002). These elements are: culture, leadership and evaluation. The CAI assesses these three elements. Each element has characteristics assessed along a continuum from 'weak' to 'strong'. For an effective culture that is receptive to change and has person-centred ways of working, the three elements all need to be 'strong'.

By completing the CAI, a team will be able to assess whether the context in their clinical setting is conductive to person-centred practice and the level of receptiveness of the context to change and development. The tool provides evidence of any changes that need to be made in order to create a strong context.

The *WCCAT* (McCormack et al., 2009a) has been informed by a number of theoretical frameworks and development processes (Table 7.1).

The use of these theoretical perspectives are illustrated in the conceptual model in Table 7.2. This model demonstrates the linkages between the different levels of culture as described by Schein (2004) (superficial, middle and deep) and how the phases of observation, reflection and feedback that underpin the WCCAT enable a deep understanding of workplace culture to be achieved and developed in a practice development action plan. The WCCAT adopts a five phase process to undertaking an observation study, analysing the data, feeding back to clinical teams and developing action plans. The five phases are:

1. *Phase 1 – Pre-observation*: This phase involves the preparation of the setting for observation and preparing the observer for the role.
2. *Phase 2 – Observation*: Observation of the workplace culture should be undertaken at the negotiated time by two trained observers using the WCCAT observation proforma. Who the observers are may be different in each project in which the

Table 7.1 Theoretical perspectives underpinning the WCCAT

Framework	Contribution to the WCCAT
The PCN Framework (McCormack & McCance, 2006)	The PCN theoretical framework has identified five care processes for patient-centred care and seven attributes of the care environment. These care processes and attributes have informed the observation foci.
Critical companionship (Titchen, 2001)	Critical companionship is a framework for developing helping relationships. It describes strategies for enabling enlightenment, empowerment and emancipation. In particular the strategies of observing, listening and questioning have informed the facilitation strategies in the WCCAT.
Culture (Schein, 2004)	Schein describes a conceptualisation of culture that moves from superficial to deeper levels of understanding. The three stages of analysis outlined in the WCCAT are based on this analysis of culture.
Workplace Culture (Manley, 2000a,b)	Manley developed a set of staff, patient and workplace indicators that she suggests need to be in place for an effective person-centred and learning culture. These have been integrated into the observation foci.
Essence of Care (Department of Health [England], 2001c)	Patient-focused benchmarks for clinical governance. Nine fundamental aspects of care derived from what patients consider important. Elements of these benchmarks have been integrated into the observation foci.

WCCAT is being used and may include different combinations of internal and external observers. Observers should maintain field notes about the experience as a process for reviewing the effectiveness of the observation undertaken.

3. *Phase 3 – Consciousness raising and problematisation*: When the observation is finished, the observers clarify with individual team members anything they are unsure of. They should also discuss with staff-specific aspects of the observation data that they want to further clarify or gain a deeper understanding of.

4. *Phase 4 – Reflection and critique*: Both observers compare their observations and agree a common set of issues to feedback to the ward team. During the feedback session, a critical dialogue is facilitated by the observers with staff. This is done by the observers presenting their 'common issues' as impressions only and putting them up to challenge by staff. Each observation area is discussed in this way and the discussion includes the comparing of the issues raised with the espoused philosophy/values and beliefs/empirical evidence.

5. *Phase 5 – Participatory analysis and action planning*: The data analysis phase should be undertaken as a participatory analysis with the ward staff. As many of the ward staff as possible, or a representative sample of staff should participate in the analysis of the data. When a finalised list of themes is achieved and agreed, an action planning workshop with the nurse leader and the staff of the clinical setting to develop an action plan is held. The processes (mechanisms) to be used to facilitate the development of PCN should also be agreed which includes an integrated evaluation framework.

Table 7.2 WCCAT conceptual model

	Culture levels (after Schein, 2004)		
	Superficial level – *What is seen* **Symbol/artefacts** Routines Actions Interactions	**Middle level** – *What is lived* **Consciousness raising and Problematisation**	**Deeper level** – *What does it mean* **Clarifying assumptions through reflection and critique**
Facilitation strategies (after Titchen, 2001)	• *Observing and listening*	• *Questioning* • *Articulation of craft knowledge*	• *Feedback* • *Challenge and support* • *Critical dialogue*
Observation areas For example, • Physical environment • Communication • Privacy and dignity • Patient involvement • Team effectiveness • Risk and safety • Organisation of care • Learning culture NB: These observation areas may change according to the context within which the WCCAT is used.	**The observers adopt the attributes, reflexivity and skills of a qualitative researcher, in observing and listening to clinicians at work in their everyday working environment.** Using the WCCAT guidelines and the observation proforma, the observer systematically records aspects of practice relevant to the focus of the observation.	**The purpose here is to check out if what has been observed matches clinicians' experience, and in so doing facilitate consciousness raising and problematisation.** Consciousness raising is a way of enabling practitioners become more alert with respect to daily practice and to their knowledge embedded in it. The observer poses questions about what has been observed, thus getting clinicians to articulate their craft knowledge. This helps the clinician to surface the tacit understandings that have grown up around repetitive and habitualised practice. Problematisation is making problematic that which had previously been assumed to be satisfactory. It may also refer to the observer pointing out or questioning things not being attended to.	**Feedback about what has been observed is offered to clinical teams using strategies of high challenge and high support as a catalyst for learning. Observers then engage clinical teams in critical dialogue with respect to this feedback.** Critical dialogue promotes collaborative interpretations, critique and evaluation of data and validates clinician's judgment (where appropriate). This fosters clinician's self-awareness, reflective and critical thinking. Challenging taken-for-granted assumptions, beliefs, values, expectations, perceptions, judgement and actions in a constructive, interested, supportive way helps clinicians gain new understandings of situations.

McCormack et al. (2009).

The conceptual framework underpinning the WCCAT enables a systematic approach to the observation of practice contexts. The observation areas are flexible and can be adapted to suit particular practice contexts. The tool relies on expert facilitators working with clinical teams to develop a programme of observation, data analysis, action planning and implementation that is collaborative, inclusive and participative.

Points to Ponder

Consider your own workplace and how you perceive PCN currently. Consider the following questions:

1. Do you have explicit shared values about PCN?
2. Do you have an explicit focus in your workplace on the continuous development of PCN?
3. What resources do you have available to you to enable you to assess your practice context using tools such as the CAI and WCCAT?
4. What support would you need to make effective use of these frameworks?

Outcomes

We have identified three outcomes that can be evaluated. However, these outcomes need to be considered alongside the enablers and contextual issues in order to demonstrate the M, C, O relationship – that is, the relationship between the mechanisms (processes, inputs) used to develop PCN, the context (the contextual issues that enable or hinder PCN to be realised) and the processes achieved.

A key premise of our PCN Framework is that nurses as care givers need to be enabled to engage with person-centred principles and operationalise these in their practice. A key consideration here is the extent to which nurses feel satisfied and involved with their work. Equally, it has been recognised that whilst there is a lot of emphasis on providing care that is person-centred, translating the core concepts into professional practice is challenging, with few research studies reported that evaluate the caring outcomes that may arise from PCN (McCormack & McCance, 2006).

Therefore, we propose the use of the 'Person-Centred Nursing Index' (PCNI) (Slater, 2006) and 'patient stories' (Hsu & McCormack, 2006) as effectives methods for evaluating the three outcomes from PCN (satisfaction with care, involvement with care, feeling of well-being).

The Person-Centred Nursing Index

The PCNI was generated from an amalgamation of key findings from an extensive systematic literature review, focus groups and a pilot study (McCormack et al., 2008). Its psychometric properties were tested and strong evidence of its validity and reliability was established (Slater, 2006). The PCNI comprises three sub-scales – 'The Nursing Context Index' (NCI) and 'The Caring Dimensions Inventory' (CDI) and 'The Nursing Dimensions Inventory' (NDI).

The NCI – A Measure of Nursing Perceptions of a Therapeutic Culture: Given the complexity of PCN, it is important that any evaluation of it takes account of each of the different attributes of PCN outcomes indicated in the outcomes framework (Figure 7.3). The NCI focuses on these attributes and how these attributes effect organisational factors such as job satisfaction, job stress and outcome variables like nurses' job commitment and intention to leave the job due to the absence of the factors that enable PCN to happen. Organisational culture research supports the link between the attributes and outcomes (Manojlovich & Laschinger, 2007; Gunnarsdóttir et al., 2009).

Research into the validity and reliability of the NCI (McCance et al., 2008) demonstrated that adequate staffing levels and nurse management were strongly related to job stress and job satisfaction. None of the organisational traits were directly related to nurses' intention to leave. However, the stress scales and job satisfaction scales were significantly related to intention to leave. Adequate staffing levels, good inter-professional relationships and effective nurse management at a unit level, (requisites of PCN) have causal links with higher job satisfaction (Manojlovich & Laschinger, 2007) and nurse burnout (Gunnarsdóttir et al., 2009).

The NCI has been shown to be a well-founded and valid measure of PCN and that it can be used to provide a picture of relationships between factors in a nurse practice environment (Slater et al., 2009).

The CDI *and* NDI: The CDI was developed by Watson and colleagues (1999, 2001). It comprises 35 operationalised statements of nursing actions designed to elicit the degree to which participants perceive these actions as representative of caring using a five-point likert scale. The items included in the instrument have been categorised as 'psychosocial', 'technical', 'professional', 'inappropriate' and unnecessary activities:

- *Technical nursing*: Items that indicate technical and professional aspects of nursing (14 items).
- *Intimacy*: Getting to know a patient and becoming involved with them (10 items).
- *Supporting*: Items that indicate helping the patients with spiritual matters (2 items).
- *Unnecessary nursing*: Aspects of nursing that are not inappropriate or unprofessional but would not normally be expected of nurses (4 items).
- *Inappropriate aspects of nursing*: Nursing actions, which, in addition to being unnecessary, are certainly not, recommended aspects of nursing (5 items).

The CDI provides data on nurses' experience of caring. The patients' experience of caring is measured using the NDI. The NDI (Watson et al., 1999) was developed to assess non-nursing views on what constitutes caring. It was based on Watson's initial work with the CDI and differed in the perspective from which caring was viewed.

It has been used to effectively assess non-nursing populations' perceptions of caring (Watson et al., 1999).

The CDI has been used to ascertain perceptions of caring from the perspective of a range of groups, including registered nurses, nursing students and non-nursing students (Watson et al., 1999, 2003a), between different clinical areas and specialities (Lea & Watson, 1995, 1999; Walsh & Dolan, 1999) and from an international perspective (Watson et al., 2003b). An evaluation of the use of the CDI and NDI by McCance et al. (2008) identified consistent scoring of 12 core statements over the 5 time points, suggesting it provides a strong indicator of nurses' perception of caring. The findings also mapped onto the PCN Framework of McCormack and McCance (2006). Mapping the core statements onto the PCN Framework reaffirms the strong correlation between caring and PCN as perceived by nurses. In relation to person-centred processes, the statements that remained consistent over time spanned across the five components presented in the PCN Framework, with none emerging stronger than any others. This reinforces the validity of the range of person-centred processes presented within the PCN Framework. The findings also highlighted the need for good communication skills and their centrality in developing therapeutic relationships.

In stark contrast with the nurses, McCance et al. (2008) found that the perception of patients on their experience of caring was variable, with very few statements remaining consistent over time. This would suggest that the promotion of a culture of person-centredness does not translate into a difference in patients' perceptions of caring. The item that was most significant was the importance of 'involving a patient in care'. This reinforces the importance of involving patients and clients in decisions made regarding their care and treatment, and thus its importance as an outcome indicator of PCN.

Patient stories

In life generally, we are recognised by our narrative identities (Gadamer, 1993), that is 'who' we are as individuals and in communities, who speaks; who acts; who recounts oneself and who is the moral subject (McCormack, 2002). So, for example, in a care situation, our narrative identity will be recognised by the various roles played out – the person being cared for, the professional carer, the family member, the cleaner, etc. Narrative is grounded in 'story'. Stories represent a holistic view of persons and are shaped and reshaped by our engagement with others. Because of the richness of stories and their holistic nature, patient story telling has become an important and accepted method of evaluating the quality of the experience of care and service delivery by patients and families (Down, 2004). In a study that focused on developing person-centred practices in a rehabilitation unit for older people, Hsu and McCormack (2006) developed a framework for collecting and analysing patient

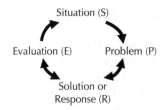

Situation (S)

Evaluation (E)   Problem (P)

Solution or
Response (R)

S: background of the narrator (patient).
P: how the past shapes perceptions of the present?
P: how the present shapes perceptions of the past?
R: how both shape perceptions of now to the future?
E: why some elements are evaluated differently from others?

Figure 7.5 The SPPRE Framework for organising narratives.

stories and translating them into service improvement plans. A three step approach to the analysis of patient stories and their translation into action plans was developed and tested in practice:

Step 1 – Organisation of narratives: This step involves organising the identified narratives into time sequences. The ordering of the narrative follows the SPPRE Framework set out in Figure 7.5.

Step 2 – Problem–solution pattern framing: Using Hoey's problem–solution pattern framework (http://www.developingteachers.com/tips/pasttips58.htm accessed May 2010) is the next step. During this step, the organised narrative is discussed to identify the problems identified by the patient/family (based on past and current perceptions), the potential range of solutions that are either directly proposed by the patient/family or that can be surmised from the story itself and the solution patterns that are revealed through the patients narrative, that is the pattern of solutions that the patient has drawn upon in the past and their future ambitions.

Steps 3 – Discussion and action: Group discussions are facilitated with teams drawing upon key questions derived from the individual patient stories and relating discussions to the PCN Framework (McCormack & McCance, 2006). Actions are identified for the development of person-centredness and mechanisms for addressing these actions identified.

Points to Ponder

Consider your own workplace and how you evaluate PCN currently. Consider the following questions:

1. Could the use of these methods enable you to demonstrate the effectiveness of your practice?
2. What support do you have available to you to enable the analysis of the data you collect?
3. What facilitation support do you have available to you?
4. What resources do you have available to you to enable you to evaluate the outcomes from your PCN developments?
5. What support would you need to make effective use of these methods?

Summary of Key Points

The literature on PCN is weak in terms of methods for evaluating outcomes, with little clarity about outcome focus, methodologies or methods. We have identified three themes for outcome measurement and suggest that PCN should be able to demonstrate outcomes in these three themes – satisfaction with care, involvement with care, feeling of well-being. Outcomes in these themes can be demonstrated from the perspectives of both staff and patients/families. We have proposed that the adoption of methodological principles derived from realistic evaluation can overcome many of the challenges associated with critiques of outcome evaluation in nursing. The adoption of these principles enables the identification of context-specific mechanisms to be identified for the development of person-centredness and the application of methods to evaluate the three outcomes arising. This approach enables a systematic articulation of process–outcome patterns and the transferability of methods to other settings through shared learning. However, what is clear is that in order for these outcomes to be achieved, a continuous participatory and inclusive developmental approach needs to be adopted in the development and evaluation of PCN.

Endnote

1. Binnie and Titchen do not refer to 'person-centredness' in their work. Instead, they use the term 'patient-centredness'. However, the principles and values underpinning the research and development work and the culture developed bear all the hallmarks of a person-centred culture and PCN.

Chapter 8

Using a Practice Development Framework to Develop Person-Centred Cultures

Introduction

Developing PCN is not a 'one-off' event. Instead it requires a sustained commitment to the facilitation of culture change in clinical settings and organisations. We have discussed pre-requisites, contextual issues and care processes in PCN, as well as the outcomes arising from the development of person-centred cultures. Whilst we have proposed a framework for evaluating person-centred outcomes, we are aware that person-centredness can still seem 'elusive' in the everyday (often chaotic) world of practice. We are also aware that many people reading this book may feel that all we are doing is 'naming that which already exists', that is 'we are doing it anyway aren't we?', whilst others may have identified issues and ideas that stimulate new ways of thinking about practice and are wondering 'how do I move towards this way of nursing?'.

We believe that many nurses in practice experience 'person-centred moments', that is, particular times in practice when everything seemed to come together and the outcome felt satisfying and rewarding. We all have memories of those moments and stories to tell of their significance to us as nurses – be it a significant event with a patient, a meaningful moment of support offered by a colleague, feedback from a leader that was intentional and empowering or an expression of thanks from a family member that made the everydayness of practice seem all worthwhile. Such 'person-centred moments' may have triggered the question, 'why can't it be like this all the time'? Whilst acknowledging that we do not work in a state of utopia and that everyday practice is challenging, often stressful, sometimes chaotic and largely unpredictable, it is important to consider how these person-centred moments can be transformed into 'person-centred cultures' of practice where satisfaction, involvement and feelings of well-being are commonplace. To do this requires a commitment to the ongoing development of practice, the paying attention to rigorous processes, the continuous evaluation of person-centred effectiveness and the celebration of successes.

In this chapter we will propose emancipatory and transformational practice development methodologies as frameworks for doing this. The philosophy and values underpinning practice development are consistent with those of person-centredness and indeed emancipatory practice development has as its primary focus 'the development of person-centred and evidence-based cultures of effectiveness'. We will describe the underpinning principles of emancipatory and transformational practice development and how these principles can be operationalised in practice. We will end with three case studies of PCN being developed through emancipatory and transformational practice development as a means of illustrating these principles and processes.

Why a Practice Development Approach?

The answer to this question is best answered by considering a letter (published with permission) from the Nurse Manager (Michelle) of a residential service for older people with mental health needs in Ireland. The manager has been participating in a programme of practice development focusing on developing person-centred practice. The 'formal' programme is about to end and she is writing to colleagues on the 'Programme Reference Group' seeking their support for sustaining the ongoing programme of work after it has formally ended.

Dear Colleagues,

In these difficult and challenging times for the health service, it may be tempting to suspend or delay the implementation of person centred care. The effort of changing culture through practice development may appear to be labour intensive and labour expensive.

I would like to make an economic case for the continuation and extension of the current programme. The [named mental health service] was fortunate to have benefited from this excellent programme for the past two years. In the beginning we were convinced that we were always person centred and that we just needed the tools and the evidence to enable us to prove it. As a manager I could see the benefit of signing up to a person centred care programme as vindication of our good intention.

I admit now that I had no idea how much we needed it. Good intention is not good practice. Residential services are largely similar in routines and rituals to that of an acute general ward. Those of us who have been patients in a hospital can identify with the unpleasant aspects of hospital life:

- Sharing a bedroom with strangers
- Sharing toilets that don't lock
- Using a commode with 3 other people in the room and a curtain protecting my privacy.
- Been woken at 6am for breakfast two hours later
- The feeling of rubber or plastic underneath the sheet

- Worry that someone can see where I have hidden my purse
- Hearing strange noise and voices in the middle of the night.

These are things that I experienced and many can identify with, but I could go home after a short time, imagine what it is like if this is forever!

I hear colleagues say 'well, you have to have a certain amount of routine or we'll never get the job done, we could be bathing all day'. What we have discovered in [practice setting] is that we too had a million different reasons why we couldn't do things differently and no reason why we should not.

To engage in person centred practice, health care workers have to stop and think and ask why are we doing certain things in certain ways; what works and what doesn't and asking residents what they would like and when. This includes looking at alternatives to rituals including bathing. Focusing on person centred practice does not take more time but does take concentrated, focused time, belief and commitment.

Nurses have given me feedback that they feel empowered by using their skills more effectively. Once established in a nurse or carer's psyche, the care process and everything involved with it becomes easier and more satisfactory for everyone concerned. I do not pretend that all staff easily adapt to person centred care and move from ritualistic practice, indeed the struggle can be great for some. I can say however, that rituals and poor practice are challenged. Residents are offered choice. The culture has shifted, and staff are open and the majority accept change.

In these challenging times staff need to be adaptable to change, which can be challenging at any time but especially so, when it is being forced because of financial constraints, which can be punitive on both staff and patients.

There exists an opportunity to use the impetus of change to implement person centred cultures. The [government change strategy] asks us to develop new ways of working and forget the silos and invisible barriers endemic in the health care system. I know now that we are better able to focus on what is important having had the benefit of emancipatory practice development. If we want to fix the big picture we must first tackle the small issues that directly effect the way we interact with patients and the resulting outcomes for them. This does not cost money but requires thought and time to reflect.

There is a general acceptance that budget cuts and reduction in staff numbers in units is inevitable given the current economic climate. Most of us can see waste in the structures and processes that result in poor value for money. As we found out in [practice setting] 'you can change the culture but you can't change the tea'! Investment in emancipatory practice development, however, represents exceptional value given its sustainability and the end result of an Effective Workplace Culture (Manley et al., 2008).

The culture cannot become effective without leadership and an understanding of what the essential elements and attributes of an effective organisation are. Manley et al. (2008) provide us with a template, emancipatory practice development with a methodology and person-centred care practices with a framework to better use the resources and skills that we have developed through this development programme.

Let us not lose the opportunity to come through these turbulent times and come out the other side with a better more focused and efficient health care environment.

Sincerely
Michelle Hardiman
Assistant Director of Nursing

Michelle's letter highlights the importance of adopting a systematic approach to the development of PCN. When we experience person-centred moments, it is easy to be seduced into thinking that is the 'norm' and lose sight of the range of experiences of patients, families and teams. A systematic and rigorous approach to practice development enables a critical reflective approach to be adopted and for everyday aspects of patient care and team relationships to be questioned, challenged and developed. Michelle also highlights the ownership of the processes and outcomes achieved among the care team and their commitment to working in this way, enabled through the facilitation approach adopted, the embracing of the processes by her (as a transformational leader), and the systematic and participator approach to the evaluation of the processes and outcomes – all characteristics of practice development.

What is Practice Development?

One of the most frequently cited definitions of practice development is:

> Practice development is a continuous process of improvement towards increased effectiveness in patient centred care. This is brought about by helping health care teams to develop their knowledge and skills and to transform the culture and context of care. It is enabled and supported by facilitators committed to systematic, rigorous continuous processes of emancipatory change that reflect the perspectives of service users.

> (Garbett & McCormack, 2002).

This definition reflects the central purpose of practice development, that of the development of patient-centred or person-centred care. It further highlights the need for development work to be undertaken rigorously and systematically, set within a continuous culture of improvement. Practice development according to this approach, differs from traditional notions of implementing evidence-based care and bringing about change in that the emphasis is not just on changing a particular practice, but also on transforming the culture(s) and context of care settings. The definition also highlights the interconnected and synergistic relationship between the development of knowledge and skills, facilitation and systematic, rigorous and continuous processes of emancipatory change in order to achieve the ultimate purpose of evidence-informed person-centred care. Thus, the key foci of practice development are:

- Increasing effectiveness in person-centred care;
- Transforming practice cultures to enable and sustain person-centred ways of working and relating;
- Adopting systematic, rigorous and continuous approaches to developing practice;
- Engaging in collaborative, inclusive and participatory facilitation relationships.

Manley and McCormack (2004) developed these foci into a model called *emancipatory practice development* (ePD). With ePD, the emphasis extends beyond the changing of specific aspects of practice, such as changing wound care treatments. ePD suggests that in order to bring about sustained development of practice, health care teams need to be enabled to transform the culture and context of practice. Thus, it is a broad view of practice development and it focuses on both getting research into practice and creating a culture of innovation and clinical effectiveness. Facilitating these processes involves cycles of reflective learning and action, so that nurses develop awareness of the need for change by identifying contradictions between what is espoused (talked about) versus the realities of practice. The process therefore takes action to change practice and refine action through reflection.

These facilitated processes help nurses remove barriers to being effective and enable person-centred cultures to be developed. This type of practice development is usually enabled by a facilitator (can be someone external to the team, a member of the team itself or a combination of the two). The facilitator creates the conditions whereby reflection, critique, collaboration, high challenge with high support and active learning can be sustained as integrated components of practice and which collectively bring about changes in the practice culture. A facilitator uses a range of skills including:

- working with values, beliefs and assumptions
- challenging contradictions
- developing moral awareness (of persons)
- focusing on the impact of the context on practice, as well as practice itself
- using self-reflection and fostering reflection in others
- enabling others to 'see the possibilities'
- fostering widening participation and collaboration by all involved
- changing practices.

Facilitators are encouraged to be creative and imaginative in their work and to enable the flourishing of others through releasing their creativity and imagination also. Person-centred cultures are characterized by their qualities that enable human flourishing. Such cultures maximise the potential of individuals for growth and development as they change the way they engage and relate with others at individual, team/group, community and societal levels. Flourishing is experienced when people achieve growth that expands their boundaries in a range of directions, for example, practical (growth in expertise), emotional, social or artistic. People are helped to flourish (grow, develop, thrive) during the change through the processes of being critical and creative, in addition to an outcome of beneficiaries of the work also flourishing. Gathering data to find out whether flourishing occurs and to make it visible to others is essential.

A more recent definition of practice development aims to make more explicit the need to be creative and imaginative in the way practice is understood and the methods used to enable meaning-ful engagement, transformation and human flourishing. In Chapter 2 we identified the need for authenticity and this definition also makes explicit the need for facilitators of person-centred cultures to be authentic in their engagement with others. Such authenticity enables the release of creative energies through the sharing of values and visions and the creation of safe spaces for nurses and others to engage in meaningful critique of practice:

> Practice development is a continuous process of developing person-centred cultures. It is enabled by facilitators who authentically engage with individuals and teams to blend personal qualities and creative imagination with practice skills and practice wisdom. The learning that occurs brings about transformations of individual and team practices. This is sustained by embedding both processes and outcomes in corporate strategy.

> (Manley et al., 2008: 9)

This definition continues to hold central the outcomes from practice development (person-centred cultures, human flourishing and effec-tive workplaces). However, it emphasises the need to blend differ-ent qualities of persons, including the creative dimension, in order to achieve effective outcomes, that is the transformation of self and work-practices. McCormack and Titchen (2006) and Titchen and McCormack (2008) propose a new methodology for transformational practice development called 'critical creativity' – a methodology that integrates the cognitive with the creative in order to bring about trans-formational change. *Transformational practice development* builds upon and extends the foundations of emancipatory practice develop-ment by placing central the idea of being creative. McCormack and Titchen (2006) set out the sub-theory of *creativity* which is seen as:

> the blending and weaving of art forms and reflexivity (critical con-sciousness) located in the critical [worldview]. Blending and weaving occur through professional artistry in order to achieve the ultimate outcome of human flourishing. Thus this theory has critical, moral and sacred dimensions.

> (McCormack & Titchen, 2006: 259)

Practical activity involves praxis through which practitioners learn how to pick out significant features of their environment, develop insightful responses to these features, and adjust and adapt them-selves to the particularities of a given situation. Of course, praxis can be informed by theory, but genuine praxis requires that practitioners go far beyond learning this theory in order to be effective practition-ers, that is we need to place ourselves in the context of theory by how we live, feel and know the environment/landscape of practice. Practitioners need to employ a kind of creative activity whereby they enable themselves to perform in particular situations. Practising this creative activity and developing practical knowing enables practition-ers to develop a professional artistry without which their interventions or transformative actions in the practical world would be clumsy, routine or unresponsive. Recently, Titchen and McCormack (2008) demonstrated how the methodology of critical creativity through the use of creative methods grounded in nature enables engagement with reflective practical action. Without such creativity, the knowing that is at the heart of transformative action cannot be fully realised through the professional artistry of practice.

We have highlighted the importance of facilitation in the development of PCN. Holistic and creative facilitation is critical to the success of emancipatory and transformational practice development. However, Titchen and McCormack (2008) argue that '. . . facilitators cannot go out and just do something to transform people, contexts or cultures and bring about human flourishing. Nor can they expect that by doing things, transformation will occur. Rather, they have to create the conditions to enable and sustain transformation and thus the potential for people to flourish.' Such conditions include the letting go of negative energies that get in the way of creativity and meaningful engagement, the creation of spaces that are free from judgement and negative critique, engaging authentically with others and having the courage to do and be 'different', experiencing stillness and contemplation, using the work-environment to experience deep reflection and re-framing of practice and finally celebrating.

Working with holistic and creative facilitation in practice development achieves outcomes of:

- A workplace culture that is person-centred, evidence-informed and enables human flourishing.
- Team structures and processes that are built upon meaningful and authentic engagement with commitment to continuous improvement of self, team, individuals and organisation.
- A commitment to work-based learning with its focus on active learning and formal systems for enabling learning in the workplace to transform care.
- Integration and enabling of both the development of evidence from practice and the use of evidence in practice.
- The blending of mind, heart and creative energies, thus enabling practitioners to free their thinking and allow opportunities for human flourishing to emerge.

The methodology of practice development creates the conditions to question existing practice and to continuously develop effectiveness in PCN. It provides a dynamic, creative and systematic approach for revealing the 'black box' that is practice context. The use of a variety of forms of evidence is the key to successful practice development and a strength of the methodology is the contextualizing of evidence so that it makes sense to those using it. Because emancipatory and transformational practice development has at their core, the development of person-centred cultures of effectiveness and the enabling of human flourishing, it provides a meaningful framework or engaging clinical teams with service users in the development of PCN.

How can Practice Development Methodology be made real in Practice?

In a concept analysis of practice development, Garbett and McCormack (2002) proposed a framework that enabled the definition of practice development to be translated into practice. We have taken that framework as a basis for understanding how to use practice development methodology to develop PCN, but have added elements of transformational practice development to it, in order to integrate both the cognitive and creative facilitation processes needed (Figure 8.1).

Using this framework is not a linear process, but instead practice developers working in this way need to adopt a reflexive approach (taking action, reflecting on action and redesigning further action based on individual and shared reflections). In our approach to practice development, having a shared vision for PCN is the starting point. Identifying the values that a team holds about person-centredness, what it means to them, what it would 'look like' in practice, and roles and responsibilities for making person-centredness a reality, begins to create a landscape for individuals and teams to explore, debate and critique. Using both cognitive processes for developing shared

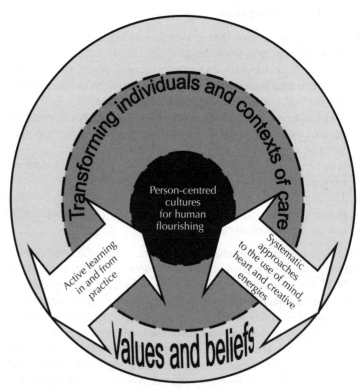

Figure 8.1 Practice development methodology (adapted from Garbett and McCormack (2002)).

values such as that developed by Warfield and Manley (1990) or creative approaches such as those described by Boomer et al. (2008) and Titchen and McCormack (2008) all help to develop a shared set of values to act as a rudder for guiding the focus of practice development work to develop more person-centredness.

Alongside developing shared values there is a need to determine how closely aligned these shared values are to existing practice, that is, a need to undertake an assessment of the practice context and the need for transformation. A variety of processes and tools can be used depending on the focus being adopted. However, the use of focus groups, creative workshops, reflective dialogues, patient stories/user narratives and critical dialogues are all useful ways of assessing the practice context and the need for change. In addition, structured processes can be used, such as the Workplace Culture Critical Analysis Tool [WCCAT] (McCormack et al., 2009), the Context Assessment Index (McCormack et al., 2008), the Person-Centred Nursing Index and the Person-Centred Caring Index [PCNI and PCCI] (Slater et al., 2006), active learning with environmental assessment and observations of practice (2008b), dementia care mapping (Kitwood & Bredin, 1992[1]), tools for facilitating systematic engagement (Walsh et al., 2005) and structured action-orientated approaches to research and evaluation, such as Appreciative Inquiry (Reed, 2007).

Assessment of the practice context provides a 'picture' of the practice setting. It enables the comparison of the 'reality of practice' with the 'espoused reality' (as articulated in the shared values). From the analysis of this information and data, an action plan can be developed.

Whilst an action plan will provide a structured framework for identifying the key issues to address in the transformational change programme, it is essential that this plan is underpinned by 'active learning' and facilitation. Dewing (2008b) describes the key characteristics of active learning as being reflection, dialogue with self and others and engaging in learning activities in the workplace that make use of the senses, multiple intelligences and doing things (i.e. workplace learning activities) collaboratively with others. In an active learning approach, all aspects of practice pose opportunities for learning and integration of new and innovative ways of practicing with reflective learning and engagement. Such active approaches to learning can be augmented and enhanced by critically creative approaches to reflection and action (McCormack & Titchen, 2006; Titchen & McCormack, 2008). Fundamental to all of this work are 'CIP Principles' (McCormack et al., 2007) – Collaboration, Inclusion and Participation. The CIP principles ensure that the development programme is owned by all staff, patients/service users and families, managers and other key stakeholders; that all perspectives are considered (even dissenting voices – Manley, 2004) and that ways of engaging focus on enabling all stakeholders to participate and feel involved.

All of these processes need to be systematically evaluated and Wilson et al. (2008) proposed a model for doing this creatively and integrated with practice development processes, called 'Praxis Evaluation'.

This approach to the development of PCN is systematic, creative, collaborative, inclusive, participatory and fun. It is an ongoing process and whilst it may have an agreed starting point it should become an integrated part of practice and be an ongoing process, all the time striving for even more person-centredness.

Case Studies of PCN Developments using Emancipatory and Transformational Approaches

A Collaborative Practice Development Programme for Clinical Nurse Leaders: 'Creating the Conditions for Growth'

Christine Boomer and Brendan McCormack, Northern Ireland[2]

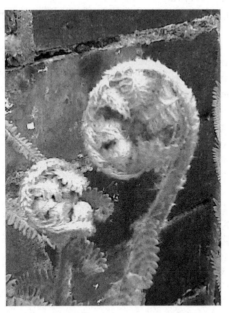

This case study will describe how a 3-year practice development programme for clinical nurse leaders utilised emancipatory practice development principles and processes as a means of developing person-centred workplace cultures. In reality, the day-to-day programme was operationalised through action research and work-based learning. For the purposes of this case study the numerous, and often complex, activities from the programme will be synthesised and subsequently mapped to the adapted practice development framework (Figure 8.2). Where applicable the relevant areas of the PCN Framework will also be highlighted *[in italics]*.

At this stage it should be stated, that although person-centredness was core to the programme, the PCN Framework was not explicitly utilised to operationalise the activities with participants as the commencement of this programme coincided with McCormack and McCance's (2006) original work on developing the PCN Framework.

The Practice Development Programme in Context

This was a 3-year collaborative practice development programme for the clinical nurse leaders (nursing unit managers) ($n = 48$)

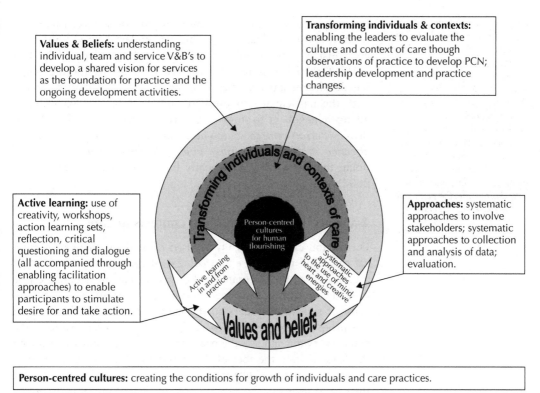

Values & Beliefs: understanding individual, team and service V&B's to develop a shared vision for services as the foundation for practice and the ongoing development activities.

Transforming individuals & contexts: enabling the leaders to evaluate the culture and context of care though observations of practice to develop PCN; leadership development and practice changes.

Active learning: use of creativity, workshops, action learning sets, reflection, critical questioning and dialogue (all accompanied through enabling facilitation approaches) to enable participants to stimulate desire for and take action.

Approaches: systematic approaches to involve stakeholders; systematic approaches to collection and analysis of data; evaluation.

Person-centred cultures: creating the conditions for growth of individuals and care practices.

Figure 8.2 Summary of the programme mapped to the practice development framework.

associated with16 units (wards/clinics) within two acute health care organisations in Northern Ireland. The focus of the programme was the development of the leadership potential of the participants and the enhancement of person-centred care practices through a series of development activities initiated and sustained by the leaders and their teams. There were three concurrently running action cycles that enabled the programme to meet its vision and aims: developing a shared vision, the context of care delivery and maximising leadership potential.

Developing person-centred nursing is like unpeeling the different layers of an onion! Each time you peel off a layer (a layer may represent non-person centred care or use of inappropriate language for example) there is always another layer underneath that we need to get stuck into. It takes resilience to get to the kind of care we want and like some of the challenges we face from colleagues, if you cut the onion in the wrong way 'it can make you cry'.

Mapping the Programme to the Practice Development Framework (Figure 8.2)

Values and beliefs

Clarifying and subsequently working with values and beliefs is a core to practice development *[and a pre-requisite of person centredness]* and hence this was the first activity undertaken by the programme participants. This involved developing vision statements

For me developing person-centred care is like playing the card game 'patience'. We have to have patience to deal with the variety of positive and negative attitudes we meet along the way. The 52 cards in the pack symbolise two things for me – the multidisciplinary team members, patients and families and also the multiple steps and stages needed in the development of person-centredness. If a card is missing, the game cannot be played to the end!

for practice (an overall programme vision, for services [the directorates] and individual units). This was undertaken with the leaders utilising values clarification (Warfield & Manley, 1990). This enabled participants to establish the foundations for the ongoing developmental activities. The programme facilitators worked with the participants to promote collaboration and inclusion of all team members to ensure the visions were both 'shared' and 'live'. [*Person-centred outcomes, clarity of values and beliefs, effective staff relationships, power sharing.*] The process for doing this work has subsequently been published (Boomer et al., 2008).

Transforming individuals and contexts of care

One action cycle specifically focused on making changes to clinical care, and the culture and context of care delivery as this was a core aim of the programme. Leadership has an irrefutable role in achieving cultural change, with cultural change being an indicator of successful leadership (Boomer et al., 2008). Therefore, in this programme the leaders (participants) were considered to be the gatekeepers to changing the practice culture and context. Although the leaders were the foci of the development activities they were expected to increase collaboration participation and inclusion with their local teams in the development of the culture of care [*power sharing, shared decision-making systems*]. A number of key processes were utilised: the use of facilitators to provide challenge and support to the participants to develop as leaders and integrate their learning into changing practice (active learning), [*developed interpersonal skills, power sharing, potential for innovation and risk-taking*]; evaluating current practice through audit, interviews with staff and patients and observation of practice (Boomer & McCormack, 2008; McCormack et al., 2009).

(Active) learning in and from practice

Initially person-centred nursing is like finding those perfect 'Jimmy Choo' shoes – they look fabulous and will solve all your fashion problems. You love them and you wear them a lot. But then they begin to pinch, the change they bring to the rest of your outfit brings uncomfortable situations and it is hard to walk with them. You want to take them off and put on your old favourites. But soon you realise that they are slowly becoming more comfortable and that these shoes really fit. 'Walk a mile in my shoes and then you will know me'.

Dewing (2008b: 273) describes active learning in the PD context as revolving 'around reflection, dialogue with self and others and engaging in learning activities in the workplace that make use of the senses, multiple intelligences and doing things (i.e. workplace learning activities) together with colleagues and others'. In this programme a number of approaches were utilised to facilitate this, the key strategy being action learning sets. There were four sets in total, each having approximately 10–12 members, comprising of a mix of grades (managers, clinical leaders, deputy clinical leaders, specialist nurses) from both participating hospital sites. These sets provided an increased opportunity for shared learning, collaboration and networking amongst the participants (McCormack et al., 2008) [*effective staff relationships, supportive organisational systems, knowing 'self'*].

Systematic approaches (to the use of mind, heart and creative energies)

Being systematic is key to practice development. This particular programme, although both large and complex, systematically evaluated practice(s), processes and development throughout the 3 years. This involved collaboration with service users (through a patient panel), key internal and external stakeholders (through an advisory group), staff (through a staff nurse panel) and participants (through site facilitators and learning sets). The use of active learning approaches by facilitators enabled participants to creatively explore their existing practice through the systematic audit and evaluation of practice (e.g. interviews with patients and staff, observations of practice), and subsequently developing action plans to enable personal and practice development.

Person-centred cultures (for human flourishing)

The development of person-centred practices was espoused in the vision developed by participants at the outset of the programme, and was either implicit or explicit in the service and unit visions. Analysis of the audit data from the 3 years alongside that from the research evaluation demonstrated that the programme had created the conditions for growth *[flourishing]*, in care practices, in individuals, team, facilitators and at service level. Examples described by patients included: team spirit, effective teamwork, friendliness and professionalism of staff, 'knowing' the patients *[feeling of well-being, professionally competent, effective relationships, satisfaction with care]*. However, this programme was the start of a journey in striving for better person-centred practice, the development continues.

Narrative Demonstrating a Participant Journey

A narrative prepared from a synthesis of feedback reflects a participant's journey during the programme, demonstrating the impact participation in practice development has on person-centredness.

Feeling isolated in my role, having received little or no induction, I came into the project nervous, apprehensive, resistant and skeptical of hidden agendas. I became exposed to lots of new 'alien' processes including reflection and action learning. I felt uncomfortable and exposed. Initially I thought my issues and problems were unique to me, but then the networks developed and the sharing began. I felt a sense of closeness with others. I started to look at myself, how I spoke to others, behaved in meetings, how I led in the ward. I learned new ways to deal with my problems and used reflection to break things down, to problem solve, look at me and my

(Continued)

role. I felt challenged in many ways; my ways of working and behaving etc, but now I feel better equipped for what I do on a daily basis. We work more as a team, we have a vision, we have challenged our practice, but change is unsettling for all. I have learned to release control and watch the team develop and flourish as a result; the ripple from lots of small changes in how we do things in the ward. Examples of which include: we took time to consider how we greet our patients and families from when they come through the door, we communicate better, our information leaflet has been improved to meet patient and relatives needs more. I feel a sense of team cohesion with my peers in the directorate/division, I no longer feel alone. This experience has pushed me more than I would have done myself and I've gone to those slightly dangerous places I wouldn't have done before. It's been worth the challenge, and the joy is the momentum that exists to keep it going, it can't stop now.

(Boomer & McCormack, 2007)

An Experience of Using a Framework for the Development of Person-Centred Practice

Lorna Peelo-Kilroe, Ireland

The PCN Framework was used in a national practice development programme to guide practice development groups to target areas for development[3]. We started using the PCN Framework (McCormack & McCance, 2006) following the first programme evaluation findings from the Person-Centred Caring Index questionnaires (PCCI), the Person-Centred Nursing Index questionnaires (PCNI) and the Context Assessment Index (CAI) questionnaires. We realised that in order to be able to interpret the findings from the questionnaires and put them into context we needed a structure. Without this we had a lot of information that we were unsure what to do with, or what it was telling us. The data from the questionnaires revealed issues regarding team work, decision-making, and some staff feeling that they couldn't influence their colleagues to change their practice because they were not 'senior enough', or that they couldn't challenge senior staff in their teams, 'it isn't done here'. We looked at the Framework when we first started the programme and were somewhat familiar with the elements, such as the pre-requisites and the care environment, but at this stage were unsure how we could incorporate the Framework into our practice development work.

The fire is taking off, what we need is a bellows of air to get the fire raging so that it can be sustained – the PCN Framework can be that bellows.

When we were reviewing the evaluation data it was suggested that we review the findings using the Framework to map common themes. We realised that there were notable themes emerging from the data that we could identify under the 'care environment' construct. The issue regarding decision-making was strongly identified in the findings from the questionnaires. The group was aware that they needed to focus on how they worked as teams, how they communicated with each other within their teams. However, this seemed somewhat vague with some group members stating that they had good team working practices and others not so. How decisions are made in teams is just one aspect of team work and can not be viewed in isolation.

We looked at the care environment aspects of the Framework and considered the findings of the questionnaires under all the areas, such as power sharing, skill mix, effective staff relationships, supportive organisational structures and opportunities for innovation. All of these areas had some bearing on the questionnaire findings. We looked at the skill mix of the teams and identified broadly the roles within the skill mix and there was some misunderstanding about roles within teams that was discussed and clarified. This was particularly useful in light of the recent development in Ireland of the 'health care assistant role', and how that fits into the skill mix of the teams. This discussion led naturally to power sharing and decision-making issues. If, at hand-over time, nurses are simply allocating tasks to the team, it does not leave any room for sharing decisions about the plan for the day. It also gives the impression that every day is the same and not planned in light of the identified care needs for that day, the available skill mix, the individual requirements of residents, activity arrangements for relatives, all of which can change from day to day.

It was identified that hand-over time needs to involve the whole team and although as always, time is limited this could still be achieved within a reasonable time frame. This created more opportunities for innovation within the teams and a greater sense of team working and communication, which helped to improve staff relationships. There was more emphasis on valuing each member of the team by giving everyone the opportunity to forward ideas, share information that contributes to planning for care and offer opportunities to challenge task-orientated care practices. This in turn contributed to developing an organisational system that focused on the care environment and reduced the attitude of 'I am just a care attendant' or 'I am just the staff nurse'.

The Framework was a very effective guide in assisting the group to challenge custom and practice and enabled a structured way of targeting specific areas for growth and development within the organisation. It is also a constructive way of planning organisational practice development based on progressing through the various sections of the Framework and mapping developments to the relevant sections. The sites involved in the national practice development programme introduced the PCN Framework, undertook structured processes and outcome evaluations at various stages of the programme, and as outlined in the example above, the Framework offers structure to the findings. Initially it was challenging to use the Framework because the relevance of each element was not always obvious. Groups felt

Developing PCN in my unit has required me to wear a 'hard hat'. I have needed to be resilient throughout the programme in order to challenge and support people effectively and 'live to tell the tale'!

that they were working effectively as teams, they had common values and beliefs about their care and that ultimately they were person-centred. Through practice development work, assumptions were challenged and slowly there was an awareness that practices previously thought to be person-centred were no longer appropriate; what was thought to be good team working was challenged through feedback exercises; and observations of care practices and general awakening of understanding about the meaning of person-centred care was becoming evident. When this started to happen, the Framework became more relevant to individuals and groups and it was then easier to identify areas of practice to develop.

Journeying from 'I have a Dream' towards 'Yes, we can': A Dialogue about leading the Development of Person-Centred Nursing

Shaun Cardiff and Marie-Louise van Hest, the Netherlands

Shaun: 'When we first met I was working for the nursing faculty of a Dutch university.'		Marie-Louise: 'I was working as a unit manager in a Dutch general hospital.'
'At first we seemed to have different dreams, but we soon realised that we both wanted to transform current nursing practice, to make it more person-centred. But would it just be a dream? This is our story.........'		

SHAUN: I work at Fontys University, Eindhoven in the Faculty of Nursing. 'The Faculty's Knowledge Centre (KC) for the Implementation and Evaluation of Evidence-Based Practice' has a motto: 'caring for evidence, evidencing care'. With a strong belief in practice development, the KC aims to, 'together with stakeholders, take on the challenge of working in innovative and systematic ways on the development of an evidence-based, person-centred culture in health care, through using creative and critical processes and, at the same time, using, testing and generating knowledge'(Cox et al., 2009).

Person-centred care was, and still is, a new concept within Dutch nursing, although there are several-related concepts in circulation. After many years of nursing and teaching I had come to see that people tended to treat others as they themselves were treated. All too often I experienced nurses being 'told' what to do, by managers, educators and doctors. Consciously and unconsciously nurses were often excluded from decisions that would directly affect their (professional) *being*. Similarly I observed nurses telling patients what to do. Consciously and unconsciously, patients were also often excluded from decisions that would affect their *being*. Seldom, if ever, did I perceive this 'deciding for the other' as a deliberate act of oppression. Advocacy and efficiency were the main arguments for these conventions. However, I cannot say that I noticed people and organisations 'flourishing' in such cultures of managerialism.

Participating in an international practice development colloquium[4], reading about person-centredness and reflecting on what I was learning and what I had experienced in the past, I came to believe that developing person-centredness was an essential step towards enabling human flourishing for all within an effective workplace culture. So, how can person-centred care be developed within a nursing unit? If people tend to treat others as they themselves are treated, what would person-centred leadership look like? Plas and Lewis (2001: 35) describe person-centred leadership as '. . . an approach to participatory management and leadership that directs as much attention to the individual as the team, requiring senior leadership to be responsible for empowering people at all levels of the organisation, and develop quality through continuous attention to organisational culture and system processes.'

Proposing to study the development of person-centredness within a nursing context I needed a research methodology that fitted with the values I was reading and hearing talked about in relation to person-centredness: equity, respect and reciprocity. Participatory Action Research (PAR) fitted the bill. Moving in action cycles of plan–act–reflect–evaluate, social realities are researched *with* participants, as opposed to performing research *on* participants. Would a facilitation strategy of high challenge and high support raise awareness and transformation of, social structures, practices and conventions that were giving rise to events that were not person-centred or enabling people to flourish?

MARIE-LOUISE: I was leading a team of nurses on an acute care of the older person unit. The unit faced the all too common problems of increasing complexity of care, high turnover of patients and tighter budgets. Tensions were high as staff felt over-worked. Although I had been a strong leader, directing developments reasonably successfully for several years, I was becoming increasingly disappointed with the lack of self-directedness, innovativeness and critical thinking within the team. They weren't flourishing. How could I lead them out of this, releasing positive energies and decentralising responsibilities? I participated in an International Practice Development School[5] that offered new tools to work with, but more importantly affirmed my ideas that I needed to develop creativity within daily practice. During a (multidisciplinary) team meeting I facilitated a guided visualisation on how people saw the future of the unit, something totally new and unexpected for the team. After clarifying some contributions we were able to use themes that emerged for the annual planning of the unit.

Although person-centredness was a new concept for us, after Shaun's proposal for a PAR study, the unit charge nurses and I felt that it connected well with the areas of development we had identified with the team, and the participatory style of doing research matched the way we were trying to move the unit forward. Actively and collectively researching person-centredness could offer us a new direction, a new opportunity, not only to transform the unit culture, but also our leadership styles.

SHAUN AND MARIE-LOUISE: Having established that person-centredness is a relational concept we decided to orientate ourselves to how current nurse–patient and nurse–leader relationships were experienced on the unit. Patient stories of care, and staff stories of leadership, were collected using narrative interviewing. Staff stories of care were also collected during some of the daily 15-minute meetings where nurses evaluate how the day is going. This way we could collect data with minimum disruption to daily practice.

The recorded interviews and storytelling sessions were transcribed word for word and represented as coherent narratives with a beginning, middle and end. The stories, especially the patient stories, made quite an impact on staff. Both nurses and leaders became aware of the contrast between how we think others perceive situations and how they themselves actually perceived them (as were expressed in the stories told). Collectively analysing the narratives posed a challenge as none of the nursing staff had any research training. Critical creative analysis workshops were designed to enable participation even though participants had not been trained or read up on narrative analysis. During the workshop participants read the stories, reflected individually on the key themes and messages emerging from the stories, and then expressed their individual interpretations creatively. Participants were then invited to share what they 'saw', 'felt' and/or 'imagined' when looking at each creative expression. Gradually common themes emerged which were discussed and agreed upon. Returning to the transcribed stories, citations were found that supported the agreed themes. The workshop evaluations were positive: it enabled active participation in narrative analysis; the more reserved people felt that they now had 'space' to share their thoughts and interpretations and the use of creativity offered a way of expressing thoughts and interpretations that were difficult to articulate verbally. Participants felt that by working collectively, aspects of stories were brought to light that may easily have been overlooked if they had only worked alone. Shared understandings were emerging.

SHAUN: Parallel to analysing stories, I facilitated a workshop to help people become familiar with the term person-centredness and the PCN Framework (McCormack & McCance, 2006). Simply translating the original framework into Dutch was not enough, people felt that the original visual presentation (see

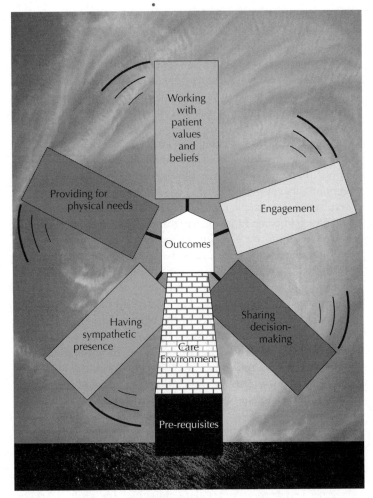

Figure 8.3 The person-centred windmill (adapted from McCormack and McCance (2006)).

McCormack & McCance, 2006) was 'too flat'. It didn't seem to radiate any message or meaning. Working with this feedback, I came up with the idea of representing the Framework as a windmill (Figure 8.3), an image that was very Dutch and may prove more appealing.

The 'sails' of the (grounded) windmill represent the five person-centred processes that need to be supported by the prerequisites and context to lift them into the 'winds' of care relationships. Each sail is a different colour (blue, purple, green, red and yellow). As the sails turn, the colours of the individual sails blend to form a white 'beacon', the outcomes.

The team agreed. They felt that this imagery brought the Framework to life, clearly demonstrating the importance of strong pre-requisites and context for person-centred processes to become active and produce results.

MARIE-LOUISE: The orientation phase involved not only the surfacing of care and leadership stories, but also learning to work collaboratively. Having Shaun as an external facilitator on the unit was both challenging and supportive for the charge nurses and myself. Shaun's presence and critical questioning during meetings caused us to stop and think about the judgements and assumptions we made, which directly affected the decisions we made.

   After 1 year we evaluated our leadership development. Once again, using creative methods, we expressed and critically reflected on our own and each others development. All three of us were becoming increasingly aware of who we were as leaders, and we were starting to think more critically before making decisions. The time had come for some structural changes.

SHAUN: To round off the orientation phase and move the team into thinking about action cycles, I made posters using the results of the critical creative analysis workshops, stories obtained from other disciplines on the unit and observations that I had made of practice and unit culture. The posters formed a kind of art gallery, a hermeneutic display of the whole and parts of the orientation phase. During a workshop team members were able to move between the whole and parts, and as they interacted with each other, claims and concerns about person-centredness on the unit emerged. Collectively we identified three areas for change: gerontological nursing knowledge; coordination and continuity of care and being critically aware of nursing/leadership practice. These became three action cycles.

SHAUN AND MARIE-LOUISE: An educational programme has been started, led by the clinical nurse specialist/case manager (who was previously one of the charge nurses). The programme is structured so as to accommodate individual and group learning, and has generally been well received. We are currently reflecting upon how to work (in a person-centred way) with some people who have had problems with the programme.

   In the second cycle we have been reviewing (and intend to transform) the nursing system. The initial phase was led by a senior staff nurse. This enabled an increase in those actively participating in the design and facilitation of action cycles. It also offered her the opportunity to develop her own leadership skills. It was her first time at leading a project so Marie-Louise supported her through this. The 'think group' consisted of various stakeholders, from a junior staff nurse to the nurse practitioner, as well as a gerontologist and the unit psychologist. After agreeing that 'coordination and continuity of care' was the main problem and goal of the review, we split into three sub-groups to design a new nursing structure and system. These three proposals were critiqued and then blended into one new proposal. Once the extra resources have been secured, we will present the proposal to the whole team for further critique and debate. The expectation is that (the team) claims, concerns and issues on the new nursing structure and system will continuously drive implementation and evaluation.

SHAUN: The third cycle is directed at developing person-centred leadership. I meet fortnightly with the clinical nurse specialist, charge nurses and Marie-Louise for 2 hours. We have been using a critical reflective inquiry structure (Kim, 1998) combined with Mezirow's (1981) levels of reflection to enable the sharing and analysis of leadership stories. There are three phases: the descriptive phase in which the story to be told is 'surfaced'; the reflective phase in which the story is reflected upon cognitively and/or creatively; and the critical/emancipatory phase in which we use what we have learnt to propose 'change for the better'. Each phase is challenging them to develop their meta-cognitive (how to think about their ways of thinking) and facilitation skills, and they are already finding themselves using these new insights and skills in their everyday leadership practice.

Once a story has been surfaced and transcribed they collectively decide either to guide the storyteller through the reflective phase, or to collectively reflect on the story facilitated by me. Although the reflection phase can be quite cognitive in nature and involve a lot of verbal communication, the use of creativity is proving extremely useful, even for the sceptics among them. For instance, we experimented with 'image theatre', taking digital photo's of 'tableau's' that we had collectively created to portray the perceived and desired situations. Downloading the photos immediately on a laptop (Figure 8.4) they were able to reflect not only on the text and personal memories of the situation, but also what they saw in the image theatre and how the actors felt whilst in position. The scope and depth of reflection increased dramatically, giving new, unexpected insights into how the situation could be interpreted and transformed.

MARIE-LOUISE: We are aware that reflecting on (person-centred) leadership alone may not be enough for sustainable change. Working with real, everyday stories has proven extremely valuable in raising awareness and motivating change. We intend to use what we have learnt about ourselves, leadership and person-centredness to facilitate nurses in the sharing of their own stories so that they too can reflect upon what it is, and what it means to be 'person-centred' on a regular, daily basis. This will be our fourth action cycle. It's too early to say exactly what form this will take. What we do know is that this will be decided together with all those leading and participating in the cycle.

SHAUN AND MARIE-LOUISE: And so we come to the end of our story, our journey so far. Using the PCN Framework/windmill as well as the tools and principles associated with emancipatory practice development, we have been critically and creatively exploring, with success, what we understand to be person-centred practice within our local context and the people we work with. As we journey, we are constantly looking for (new)

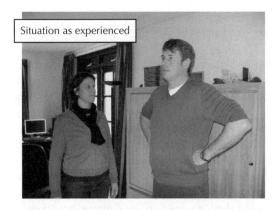

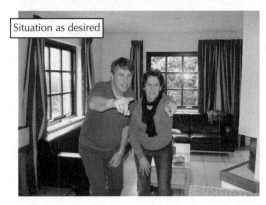

Figure 8.4 Using digital photography to capture images for immediate (collective) reflection.

ways to develop an effective, person-centred workplace culture where each and every one of us is valued as an individual and group member. What seemed a dream, of transforming leadership and nursing practice, is becoming a reality. If you were to ask us now: 'Can you?' our answer would be: 'Yes, we can.'

The Belfast Health and Social Care Trust Person-Centred Care Programme

Bernadette Gribben and Tanya McCance

Introduction

The Person-Centred Care Programme is a learning and development programme taking place within the Belfast Health and Social Care Trust. The Trust is the largest provider of health and care within Northern Ireland, delivering a range of services across four acute hospital sites and two community patches. The Trust employs approximately 9000 nurses and midwives, and is committed to the development of this workforce as reflected in organisational priorities and in our Nursing and Midwifery Strategy, *Striking the Balance* (BHSCT, 2009). The Person-Centred Care (PCC) Programme is one component in a plan of work that aims to promote effective person-centred cultures, in order to enhance the care experience of patients, clients, families and carers.

The Programme

The overarching aim of the PCC Programme is to enable nursing and midwifery teams to explore the concept of person-centredness within their own setting and to improve care delivery. The rationale for this Programme reflects the context provided in Chapter 1, and its delivery is underpinned by the principles of practice development and uses a range of practice development methods that focus on working collectively, facilitating change and evaluating practice, as described earlier in this chapter. The Programme comprises facilitated activities that focus on four consecutive themes. *Theme 1* focuses on promoting an awareness and understanding of person-centredness and reflects the challenge that at a level of principle understanding is good, but operationalising and recognising it in practice is inherently more difficult. *Theme 2* focuses on developing a shared vision, which is fundamental to a practice development approach. The rationale for this activity is based on the premise that by making assumptions conscious, explicit value and beliefs can be articulated (Manley, 2000b), which is crucial in shaping a vision for nursing practice. *Theme 3* focuses on activities that use a range of methods aimed at collecting information on the quality of the user experience, in order to benchmark practice against the vision. This benchmarking activity informs the identification of areas for practice change, which become the focus for *Theme 4*. The activities within each theme are presented in Figure 8.5.

Also, in order to determine the impact of the Programme, realistic evaluation is being used, which consists of cycles of evaluation. This involves patient stories, participant focus groups and the use of fourth generation evaluation (Guba & Lincoln, 1989), an approach that makes repeated use of claims (favourable assertions about the topic and its implementation), concerns (unfavourable assertions about the topic and its implementation), and issues (questions that reflect what any reasonable person might ask about the topic and its implementation).

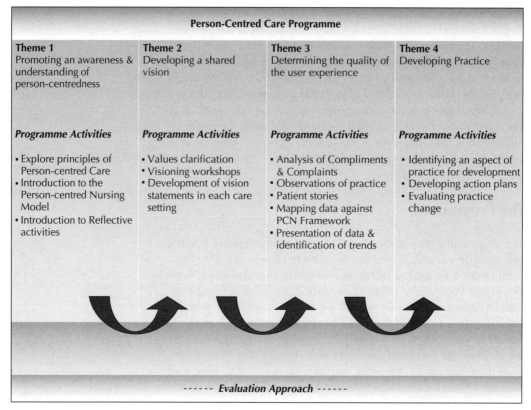

Figure 8.5 Overview of the PCC Programme.

The Participants

There are 10 participating sites from across the Belfast Health and Social Care Trust involved in the PCC Programme. All participants are working across the four hospital sites within the Trust and represent a diverse range of practice settings. Specialties include: an intensive care unit, chest medicine, cardiology intervention, a cancer unit, medicine/respiratory, mental health, eyes and ENT theatre, medical/hepatology, neurology and a brain injury unit. Each site is supported by the associated Nursing Development Lead (NDL), whose role is to support the ward managers in the implementation of the Programme.

Using the PCN Framework

The PCN Framework underpins the delivery of the Programme and is used in a variety of ways, as described below, to facilitate engagement of participants with the concept of person-centredness as it relates to their practice.

1. Using the Framework to raise awareness of the concept of person-centredness and to facilitate the development of a ward or department's shared vision.
2. Using the Framework 'in action' within the workplace as a tool to evaluate care, for example, during handover or to analyse critical events, both positive or negative.
3. Using the Framework to assess the experience of patients being cared for in each site, for example, by making sense of feedback received from compliments and complaints.
4. Using the Framework to guide the process of data analysis for the realistic evaluation. It serves as an analytical framework that enables the theming of data and the identification of possible relationships between constructs that will be crucial for testing through further research.

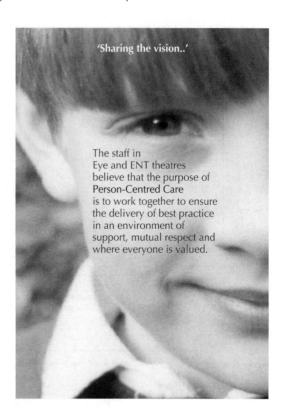

'Sharing the vision..'

The staff in Eye and ENT theatres believe that the purpose of Person-Centred Care is to work together to ensure the delivery of best practice in an environment of support, mutual respect and where everyone is valued.

The thank you letter presented below was received by one of the participating sites during the PCC Programme and was used to map against the PCN Framework. Figure 8.6 presents the outcomes from this activity. This feedback enabled staff to reflect on their practice and to recognise and celebrate how they were delivering care that was person-centred.

Dear Sr

I wish to take this opportunity to thank you and all the nursing staff on your ward for all your devotion and nursing care that I received during my stay prior to my transplant.

I can not praise you and the nursing staff enough for your kindness towards myself and members of my family, I have no doubt in my mind that without the skills of the doctors and nursing staff, I would not be in a position to write to you today.

I have never felt better for a long number of years as I do today, please convey my thanks to all the doctors and nurses on the ward for their skill and devotion. I know I have made many friends during my stay and I hope to call and see you all soon.

Once again my heart felt thanks to you all for your devotion and kindness during my stay on your ward.

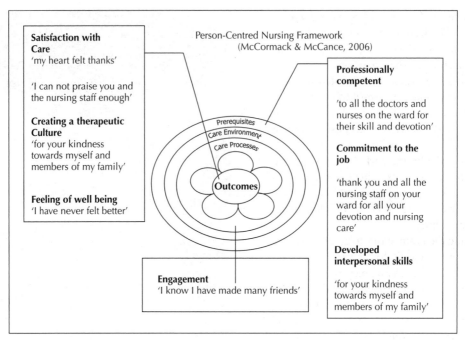

Figure 8.6 Using the PCN Framework to map compliments.

We are still on a journey within the Belfast Trust, but participants within the Programme are beginning to recognise the value of using the Framework and the potential benefits for practice, as evidenced from the experiences of our Programme participants.

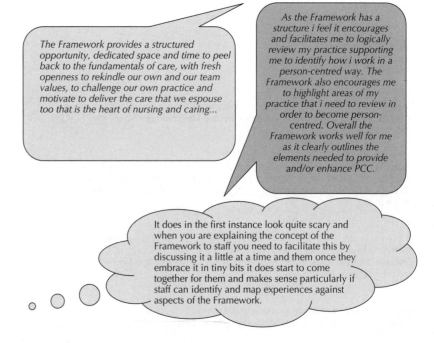

Person-Centred Practice at Uniting Care Ageing, New South Wales, Australia

Jan Dewing, Program Lead, Visiting Professor, School of Nursing, Midwifery and Indigenous Health, University of Wollongong; **Heidi Dowse,** *Learning and Development Manager, UnitingCare Ageing, South Eastern Region;* **Philip Eldridge,** *Regional Coordinating Chaplain, UnitingCare Ageing, South East Region;* **Julie Farmer,** *Regional ACFI Coordinator, UnitingCare Ageing, South Eastern;* **Tamra MacLeod,** *Nurse Practitioner, UnitingCare Ageing, South Eastern Region;* **Carmel Gibbons,** *Group Manager, UnitingCare Ageing, Mirinjani Village;* **Anna-Marie Harmon,** *Manager, Business Systems, UnitingCare Ageing, South Eastern Region.*

> Practice Development, what is that?
> Is it just about wearing another hat?
> We've tried Eden, Spark of Life, Torch Bearers and more
> Hopefully Practice Development isn't a bore
>
> The program is called 'Aspire to Inspire'
> Which sounds like all we desire
> Creativity, active learning with workplace activities
> Program days, how will we fit in that?
> Add feathers, paints, candles and coloured mats
> Hope this doesn't mean wearing a funny hat!
>
> The staff are engaged
> And the learning has begun
> We'll wait to see how much fun ....
>
> (Poem composed by Tamra)

Introduction

We have constructed a 'virtual' conversation' as our conversation did indeed take place through email from one side of the world to the other. The team and the organisation (Uniting Care Ageing South East Region Australia) have recently begun a 2-year practice development programme across all their aged care services in the region (New South Wales (NSW) and Australian Capital Territory (ACT). Taking part in this conversation are Heidi, Philip, Anna-Marie, Julie, Tamra and Carmel. Our other two team members send their apologies as they weren't able to participate.

The Conversation

JAN: *If I asked you how you envision the Person-centred Nursing Framework working in your organisation what would be your feelings and thoughts?*

HEIDI: My initial thoughts are that the PCN Framework is a comprehensive framework that once understood becomes easily applicable to a workplace. When Julie and I introduced the Framework to staff, many of them felt it was easily understood and encompassed the components of person-centred care that had been missing in the past. Staff quickly came to the realisation that previous work on person-centred care was all outcome driven. This Framework, they said, made sense to them.

PHILIP: I feel our organisation is planning for a future where the people we serve and their carers will want more choice and involvement in their care experience with us. Our future will be one where people receive person-centred care in a range of accommodation settings. The PCN Framework, which is at the heart of the 'Aspire to Inspire' Practice Development Programme, speaks directly to these aspirations and my hope is that it will provide the skeleton which will support the flesh of person-centred care in this region of the organisation. I feel that, just as a chain is only as strong as its weakest link, this hope will only be realised if each component of the Framework is seen as an integral part of the whole and given equal weight by both staff and management.

JAN: *What do you feel the PCN Framework can offer?*

HEIDI: The PCN Framework helps staff to see what it is they need to work on. It seems to be enabling our staff to hold the mirror up to themselves, their practice and workplace culture. When combined with critical reflection and active learning, staff feel empowered to change the way they work. The Framework provides a systematic and structured model to work with. When discussing the Framework with staff they comment that the Framework may not be easy to explain to others at first, but recognise that it is all encompassing. It considers processes and outcomes for older people, staff attributes and the contribution managers and leaders need to make.

JAN: *What feelings and thoughts do you have about the relationship between the PCN Framework and the Practice Development Framework?*

ANNA-MARIE: If I am completely honest I am still somewhat bewildered, confused, excited and nervous. All these feelings seem to be rolled up in one big knot that is sitting in my stomach. We delivered our first practice development day recently. Yes, I think it was successful. By successful I mean participants were more than honest in what they thought of the programme and us as facilitators. The work required to prepare for this day was considerable. I could not understand all the activities and how it all worked together. But after some considerable time it became clearer.

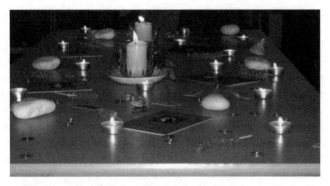

Figure 8.7 Our 'set-up' for the practice development work.

We set the room up and felt that this worked really well. The general comments from the participants ranged from 'we have walked into a wake' to 'how relaxing and beautiful it felt and looked' (Figure 8.7).

The day was a challenging one in that we had a diverse mix of participants from all work and cultural backgrounds. As we had started the day with an activity called 'Personal Weather Forecast' so too did we finish the day with this activity. What was exciting was the difference in the words expressed from the morning to the afternoon. Participants left very excited about the Framework and workplace activities . . . so much so that we struggled to keep them quiet whilst trying to explain the process to them.

Overall, it was a day of roller coaster emotions and challenges and I have no illusions that we have our work cut out for us as we work to implement the Framework and a practice development culture.

JULIE: What I felt and heard on our first programme day, were the voices of our staff, with hope, the freedom to speak, asking: 'can we make this better?' And I think because I have been reading the transformational leadership material, I tried to link cause and effect without blame; the direct correlation of information is astounding. So practice development and the PCN Framework are actually so timely for us. Innovation starts with a good idea; but this good idea will become much more than that for us. Practice development will enable and empower our staff to not only give good care; but will help our staff to value and understand themselves as people. On our first programme day Heidi and I were amazed . . . it birthed voices that identified the following snapshots for potential.

- Residents will benefit
- Staff will benefit
- You can voice your concerns in this workplace
- An opportunity to identify things that aren't working well and learn
- People are listening to us.

It is going to be a long journey of change, but very timely for all of us.

HEIDI: I believe this Framework has provided our organisation with the missing link. It has given hope to us all, that finally, person-centred care will be embedded in our culture. In the 'Aspire to Inspire Programme', the programme team aim to facilitate staff to work with all the themes of the PCN Framework starting with the pre-requisites. We are ensuring that learning about person-centredness and the Framework are connected and that this primarily takes place in the workplace and in every day practice.

JAN: *Carmel, I see you have made a contribution in prose. . . . . . .*

CARMEL: Yes, it's about that first day with the regional office staff who were included in the practice development programme. Here goes. . . .

The first day to begin our journey in Practice Development
with the staff at Regional office and Gerringong
We knew the commitment was two years and for some this
would be long
To explain the Framework was the challenge here and relate
it to the journey we were on.
The circles and the flower showed the connections and out-
comes were understood
But staff were unsure how they would get there and if the
linkages could lead to culture change
Slowly but surely as a team is the only way to arrange
An engagement of all to participate and change

The prerequisites were tied to job descriptions, Uniting Care
values and self reflection.
Staff began to understand the importance of knowing self in
order to influence others in the new direction.
The care environment was discussed at length with a potential for innovation and taking risk Some trepidation was felt
by all and this is where facilitators and meetings comes in
To support, empower participants and engage managers to
listen, not obstruct and hopefully grin
Appropriate skill mix could be addressed at recruitment
time, with education and who would fit best

Care processes was the next up for discussion
Engagement was considered most important by everyone
How to get staff on the journey with them and activities
around having fun
Proved to be the most popular one
Regional staff were tougher than expected
With questions about how it all related.
We explored ways for the staff to connect with residents in
the homes in a meaningful way

And have decided participating activity could work at the
end of the day
Some would have contact via the phone and even the lan-
guage used could have sympathetic presence
For many of the staff and residents
Providing for physical needs by care staff was understood
As Jane and I knew it would
Sharing decision making and respecting residents beliefs at
all times reflected with care plans, language and listening
and that would be fine.

Outcomes was last to be described and we all believed it
could happen
And with hard work and support we would achieve
satisfaction
With care, involvement with care, wellbeing and a therapeutic
culture for all
What we don't want to happen is to stall
Or lose momentum on this journey; it needs to be embedded
in everyday
So Uniting Care South Eastern Region can lead the way

Staff understood the outcomes well but how to get there was
not so clear
They believed it might challenge beliefs held dear

The challenge was to engage and connect with people we did
not really know
And assist them and us to learn and to grow
On both first days we set the scene with candles and rocks
and the seasons of the year
In the hopes to reach the staff differently and get them to
hear
We were unsure if we could explain and if the message would
be clear
We were learning and very nervous too
Could we deliver the message and sound true blue
Jane took the lead and I followed on
And suddenly we all started to bond
Building relationships was what we were about
And honesty helped an enormous amount.

We discussed language used at work
And this prompted a lot of talk
Combining the two groups is our next mission
And on goes the journey towards our vision
If we are going to create a culture of questioning things
And assist to empower the staff we hope that will bring
About change to current practice doesn't that have a nice
ring?

JAN: To summarise, I'm hearing that the PCN Framework feels like a comprehensive framework for developing a person-centred culture. It intuitively makes sense – it feels right. Also it is equally applicable to staff and managers. It needs to be used within practice development processes and systems to help implementation and workplace culture changes needed to ensure the Framework is adopted to its full potential. All of the themes need to be attended to. It is demanding of individuals, teams and managers in that it needs vision/aspiration along with personal courage and inspiration to achieve successful implementation.

Thank you all.

Summary of Key Points

In this chapter we have shown how the PCN Framework can be used as a practical and systematic framework for guiding the development of person-centred cultures. The stories, dialogues and creative illustrations of the experiences of both using the Framework and the adoption of a practice development approach help to bring to life what can sometimes feel like the sterile application of theory to practice. What is clear to us is that whilst the PCN Framework may be grounded in (complex) theory, it cannot be used as a 'bolted-on' theoretical framework. When the Framework is engaged within a critical reflective way then each of the constructs and the items contained within them start to act as a focus for challenging established 'ways of being' and identification of potential changes in a culture. The unraveling of one construct leads to the questioning of others and the development of an ongoing and never-ending programme of person-centred development.

Developing PCN has been like a journey for us. Some stages of the journey have been rough and some have been smooth. It has been a bit like a bus trip, collecting as many people as possible on the way and trying to get them to stay for the full experience and not get off too early. A driver (leader) is needed to keep the bus on the right route but everyone else on board needs to let the driver know where they want to go and support each other in getting there.

Developing person-centred cultures is not a one man/woman job and it is clear that it requires commitment from a whole team. Whether you are focused on PCN or a more multi-professional idea of person-centred practice the frameworks, methods and processes offered in this book provide useful components of a 'map' for guiding you on the way. We know that person-centred cultures are not achieved from one-off change events, but we also know that once a commitment to developing person-cultures is made then teams need to be able to see 'bite-sized' tangible changes to maintain commitment, enthusiasm and morale. All of the stories of person-centred culture development highlight the participatory, collaborative and inclusive nature of the processes involved and the complexity of the change processes necessary.

Progression by Mary Kinnaird, Staff Nurse, St. John's Hospital Enniscorthy, Ireland

I often hear stories of years ago,
Of regular back rounds
And sudo [sudocream] a flow.
Of lines of patients, sat on commodes,

For bath day was a day to behold.
I think to myself, what would the patient say,
If they could tell us now
About that infamous MONDAY!!

Then I wonder in awe. I sit and debate,
Are we really any better than those days of late.
Are patients got up at 07:10
Does the morning round still have to finish
Before 10.
Are patients still sat in a clumsy big chair
At unpainted walls, to sit and stare.

I take in a breath, then sigh with relief,
Those days are now gone, all be it brief.
The roughly painted walls may still be there,
But need for stimulation we are more aware.
Exercise classes are now in place, music sessions
Liven up the place.
Rarely now, do we hear people say,
Is Jane Doe for up today?
As many well know, the answer is clear,
Ask Jane Doe, she's lying right there.

We're still far from perfect, there is no fear,
We still have a long way to go from here.
But what we have now, and must strive to maintain.
Is the patient's right to choice and their right to complain.
There is a lot there to guide us.
Person centred we must stay.
And don't forget that HIQA[6], is on it's way.
And if that doesn't steer you, may I just say.
That, the patient, might be you or yours some day.

Endnotes

1. A comprehensive list of resources relating to dementia care mapping can be found at http://www.brad.ac.uk/health/dementia/dcm/publications/index.php

2. The photograph at the beginning of this case study is that of a 'Koru'. The Koru is the Māori name given to the new unfurling fern frond and symbolizes new life, growth, strength and peace. In the development of the work presented in this case study, the Koru was used as a unifying symbol for analysing the experiences of participants and the journey towards 'creating the conditions for growth'.

3. The Older Person's National Practice Development Programme is a 2-year programme of development and research work funded by the National Council for the Professional Development of Nursing and Midwifery and the Health Service Executive's Nursing and Midwifery Planning and Development Units in the Republic of Ireland. The development work focused on 20 residential units for older people and incorporated a collaborative internal and external facilitation model.

4. The International Practice Development Colloquium (IPDC) is a cooperative inquiry of practice developers and researchers from the United Kingdom, Ireland, the Netherlands, Australia and New Zealand who have focused on developing theoretical and methodological frameworks to guide practice development, participatory and practitioner research activities.

5. The International Practice Development Schools are delivered annually through the IPDC in all of the participating countries. This is a 5-day programme that enables participants to explore different aspects of person-centredness and its development through practice development methodologies.

6. Health Information and Quality Authority (HIQA), in the Republic of Ireland, is an independent agency established by the Irish Government as part of its health and social care reform programme. Its remit is to drive quality, safety, accountability and the best use of resources in the health and social care services, whether delivered by public, voluntary or private bodies. Recently HIQA have developed National Quality Standards for Residential Services for Older People.

References

Adair, J. (1987). *Effective Teambuilding*. London: Pan Books.

Adams, A. & Bond, S. (1997). Clinical specialty and organizational features of acute hospital wards. *Journal of Advanced Nursing*, 26, 1158–1167.

Adams, T. (1996). Kitwood's approach to dementia and dementia care: a critical but appreciative review. *Journal of Advanced Nursing*, 23, 948–953.

Agich, G.J. (1993). *Autonomy and Long-Term Care*. Oxford; Oxford University Press.

Aiken, H.K., Clarke, S.P., Sloane, D.M., Sochalski, J.A., Busse, R., Clarke, H., Giovannetti, P., Hunt, J., Rafferty, A.M. & Shamian, J. (2001). Nurses reports on hospital are in five countries. *Health Affairs*, 20(3), 45–53.

Aiken, L., Smith, H. & Lake, E. (1994). Lower mediare mortality among a set of hospitals known for good nursing are. *Medical Are*, 32(8), 771–787.

Aiken, L.H. & Fagin, C.M. (1997). Evaluating the consequences of hospital restructuring – preface. *Medical Care*, 35(10), OS1–OS4.

Aiken, L.H. & Sloane, D.M. (1997a). Effects of organizational innovations in AIDS care on burnout among urban hospital nurses. *Work and Occupations*, 24(4), 453–477.

Aiken, L.H. & Sloane, D.M. (1997b). Effects of specialization and client differentiation on the status of nurses: the case of AIDS. *Journal of Health and Social Behavior*, 38(3), 203–222.

Aiken, L.H. & Sochalski, J. (1997). Hospital restructuring in North America and Europe: patients outcomes and workforce implications. *Medical Care*, 35(10), NS6–NS18.

Aiken, L.H., Sloane, D.M. & Lake, E.T. (1997). Satisfaction with inpatient acquired immunodeficiency syndrome care – a national comparison of dedicated and scattered-bed units. *Medical Care*, 35(9), 948–962.

Aiken, L.H., Clarke, S.P. & Sloane, D.M. (2000). Hospital restructuring – does it adversely affect care and outcomes? *Journal of Nursing Administration*, 30(10), 457–465.

Anderson, R. (1982). *On Being Human – Essays in Theological Anthropology*. Grand Rapids: Eerdmans.

Andrews, G. (2003). Locating a geography of nursing: space, place and the progress of geographical thought. *Nursing Philosophy*, 4(3), 231–248.

Arneill, B. & Frasca-Beaulieu, F. (2003). Healing Environments: Architecture and Design Conducive to Health. In S.B. Frampton, L. Gilpin & P.A.

Charmel (Eds), *Putting Patients First: Designing and Practicing Patient-Centred Care*. San Francisco, CA: Jossey-Bass.

Baillie, L. (1996). A phenomenological study of the concept of empathy. *Journal of Advanced Nursing*, 24, 1300–1308.

Baldwin, T. (Ed.) (2004). *Maurice Merleau-Ponty: Basic Writings*. London: Routledge.

Barker, E.M. (1991). Rethinking Family Loyalties. In N.S. Jecker (Ed.) *Aging and Ethics*. Clifton, New Jersey: Humana Press.

Barker, P. (2001). The tidal model: a radical approach to person-centred care. *Perspectives in Psychiatric Care*, 37(2), 233–240.

Barker, P. (2002). The tidal model: the healing potential of metaphor within the patient's narrative. *Journal of Psychosocial Nursing*, 40(7), 42–50.

Bass, B.M. (1985). *Leadership and Performance Beyond Expectations*. New York: Free Press.

Bate, P. (1994). *Strategies for Cultural Change*. Oxford: Butterworth Heinemann.

Baumann, S.L. (2006). What does nursing practice mean? *Nursing Science Quarterly*, 19, 259–260.

Beauchamp, T.L. & Walters, L. (1989). *Contemporary Issues in Bioethics*, 3rd Edn. Belmont, California: Wadsworth Publishing Company.

Belfast Health & Social Care Trust (BHSCT) (2009). *Striking the Balance: Nursing & Midwifery Strategy 2009–2012*. Belfast: BHSCT.

Benner, P. (1984). *From Novice to Expert: Excellence and Power in Clinical Nursing Practice*. California: Addison-Wesley Publishing Company.

Benner, P. & Wrubel, J. (1989). *The Primacy of Caring: Stress and Coping in Health and Illness*. Wokingham: Addison-Wesley Publishing Company.

Berlin, I. (1992). *Four Essays on Liberty*. Oxford: Oxford University Press.

Binnie, A. & Titchen, A. (1999). *Freedom to Practise: The Development of Patient-centred Nursing*. Oxford: Elsevier.

Bishop, V. (1998). *Clinical Supervision in Practice. Some Questions, Answers and Guidelines*. Basingstoke: Macmillan.

Blegen, M.A. (1993). Nurses job-satisfaction – a meta-analysis of related variables. *Nursing Research*, 42(1), 36–41.

Blegen, M.A., Goode, C.J. & Reed, L. (1998). Nurse Staffing and Patient Outcomes. *Nursing Research*, 47(1), 43–50.

Blum, L.A. (1982). *Friendship, Altruism and Morality*. London: Routledge & Kegan Paul.

Bolan, D.S. & Bolan, D.S. (1994). A reconceptualization and analysis of organizational culture: the influence of groups and their idiocultures. *Journal of Managerial Psychology*, 9(5), 22–27.

Boomer, C. & McCormack, B. (2007). Creating the conditions for growth. Report on the Belfast City hospital and The Royal Hospitals Collaborative Practice Development Programme. Unpublished Report.

Boomer, C. & McCormack, B. (2008). 'Where are we now?' A process for evaluating the context of care in practice development. *Practice Development in Health Care*, 7(3), 123–133.

Boomer, C., Devlin, M. & McCormack, B. (2006). *Shifting the Culture of Practice: Report on the Evaluation of Pilot 1b of REACH: A Clinical Careers Framework for Nurses*. Belfast: Royal Hospitals Trust and Royal College of Nursing.

Boomer, C., Collin, I. & McCormack, B. (2008). I have a dream: a process for visioning in practice development. *Practice Development in Healthcare*, 7(2), 70–78.

Borrill, C.S., Carletta, J., Carter, A.J., Dawson, F., Garrod, S., Rees, A., Richards, A., Shapiro, D. & West, M.A. (1999). *The Effectiveness of Health Care Teams in the National Health Service.* Aston: University of Aston.

Bowling, A. (2005). *Measuring Health: A Review of Quality of Life Measurement Scales.* England: Open University Press, Maidenhead.

Boykin, A. & Schoenhofer, S. (1993). *Nursing as Caring: A Model for Transforming Practice.* New York: National League for Nursing Press.

Bradbury-Jones, C., Sambrook, S. & Irvine, F. (2008). Power and empowerment in nursing: a fourth theoretical approach. *Journal of Advanced Nursing,* 62(2), 258–266.

Brilowski, G.A. & Wendler, M.C. (2005). An evolutionary concept analysis of caring. *Journal of Advanced Nursing,* 50(6), 641–650.

Brooker, D. (2002). Dementia care mapping: a look at its past, present and future. *Journal of Dementia Care,* 10(3), 33–36.

Brown, A. (1998). *Organisational Culture,* 2nd Edn. London: Pitman Publishing.

Brown, D. (2008). Facilitating Changes in the Practice Context: Using Action Research to Uncover the Significance of Psychological Safety – An Example from Pain Management with Older People. Unpublished PhD Thesis, University of Ulster, Jordanstown, Northern Ireland.

Brown, D. & McCormack, B. (2006). Determining factors that have an impact upon effective evidence-based pain management with older people, following colorectal surgery: an ethnographic study. *Journal of Clinical Nursing,* 15(10), 1211–1351.

Brown, J., Kitson, A.L. & McKnight, T. (1997). *Challenges in Caring: Explorations in Nursing and Ethics.* London: Chapman and Hall.

Brown, L. (1986). The experience of care: patient perspectives. *Topics of Clinical Nursing,* 8, 56–62.

Brykczynska, G. (1997). A Brief Overview of the Epistemology of Caring. In G. Brykczynska & M. Jolley (Eds), *Caring: The Compassion and Wisdom of Nursing* (pp. 1–9). London: Arnold.

Buber, M. (1958). *I and thou.* Edinburgh: T Clarke.

Buber, M. (1984). *I and Thou.* Edinburgh: T & T Clark.

Buchanan, A.E. & Brock, D.W. (1989). *Deciding for Others: The Ethics of Surrogate Decision Making.* Cambridge: Cambridge University Press.

Burnard, P. (1988). Empathy: the key to understanding. *The Professional Nurse,* 3(10), 388–391.

Calman, L. (2006). Patients' views of nurses' competence. *Nurse Education Today,* 26, 719–725.

Campbell, A.V. (1984). *Moderated Love: A Theology of Professional Care.* London: SPCK.

Carper, B.A. (1978). Fundamental Patterns of Knowing. In L.H. Nicoll (Ed.) *Perspectives on Nursing Theory* (pp. 247–254). Philadelphia: J.B. Lippincott Company.

Chang, M.-Y., Chen, C.-H. & Huang, K.-F. (2008). Effects of music therapy on psychological health of women during pregnancy. *Journal of Clinical Nursing,* 17(19), 2580–2587.

Chipman, Y. (1991). Caring: its meaning and place in the practice of nursing. *Journal of Nursing Education,* 30, 171–175.

Christman, J. (1989). Introduction. In J. Christman (Ed.), *The Inner Citadel: Essays on Individual Autonomy.* Oxford: Oxford University Press.

Clarke, A. (2000). Using biography to enhance the nursing care of older people. *British Journal of Nursing,* 9(7), 429–433.

Clarke, A. (2001). *Learning Organizations, What They Are and How to Become One*. Leicester: The National Organisation for Adult Learning (NIACE).

Clarke, A., Hanson, E.J. & Ross, H. (2003). Seeing the person behind the patient: enhancing the care of older people using a biographical approach. *Journal of Clinical Nursing*, 12, 697–706.

Coeling, H. & Simms, L. (1993). Facilitating innovation at the nursing unit level through cultural assessment, part 1: how to keep management ideas from falling on deaf ears. *Journal of Nursing Administration*, 23, 46–53.

Conway, J. (1996). *Nursing Expertise and Advanced Practice*. Dinton, UK: Quay Books.

Cox, K. (2003). The effects of intrapersonal, intragroup, and intergroup conflict on team performance effectiveness and work satisfaction. *Nursing Administration Quarterly*, 27, 152–163.

Cox, K., Titchen, A., Bers, M., Cardiff, S., Legius, M. & Munten, G. (2009). Knowledge Centre Vision Statement. Retrieved 28 April, 2009, from http://www.fontys.nl/ebp/vision.statement.270167.htm

Cunningham, G. & Kitson, A. (2000a). An evaluation of the RCN Clinical Leadership Development Programme: Part 1. *Nursing Standard*, 15(12), 34–37.

Cunningham, G. & Kitson, A. (2000b). An evaluation of the RCN Clinical Leadership Development Programme: Part 2. *Nursing Standard*, 15(13), 36–39.

Cunningham, G. & Kitson, A. (2000c). An evaluation of the RCN Clinical Development Programme: part 2. *Nursing Standard*, 15(13–15), 34–40.

Cutliffe, J.R. & Wieck, K.L. (2008). Salvation or damnation: deconstructing nursing's aspirations to professional status. *Journal of Nursing Management*, 16, 499–507.

Davies, H., Nutley, S. & Mannion, R. (2000). Organisational culture and quality of health care. *Quality in Health Care*, 9(2), 111–119.

Dementia Services Development Centre (2007). *Best Practice in Design for People with Dementia*. Stirling, Scotland: Dementia Services Development Centre.

Department of Health (2006). *'Dignity in care' public survey*. London: DoH.

Department of Health [England] (2001a). *The National Service Framework for Older People*. London: Department of Health http://www.dh.gov.uk/en/Publicationsandstatistics/Publications/PublicationsPolicyAndGuidance/DH_4003066 (accessed April 2009).

Department of Health [England] (2001b). *The Expert Patient: A New Approach to Chronic Disease Management for the 21st Century*. London: Department of Health.

Department of Health [England] (2001c). *Essence of Care: Patient Focused Benchmarks for Clinical Governance*. London: Department of Health.

Department of Health [England] (2005). *Supporting People with Long Term Conditions: Liberating the Talents of Nurses Who Care for People with Long Term Conditions*. London: Department of Health.

Department of Health [England] (2007). *Putting People First: A Shared Vision and Commitment to the Transformation of Adult Social Care*. London: Department of Health.

Department of Health and Social Service and Public Safety (2008). *Improving the Patient and Client Experience*. DHSSPS: Belfast.

Dewey, J. (2004). *Democracy and Education*. Whitefish, MT: Kessinger.

Dewing, J. (2002). From ritual to relationship: a person-centred approach to consent in qualitative research with older people who have a dementia. *Dementia*, 1(2), 157–171.

Dewing, J. (2004). Concerns relating to the application of frameworks to promote person-centredness in nursing with older people. *International Journal of Older People Nursing*, 13(3a), 39–44.

Dewing, J. (2007). An Exploration of Wandering in Older Persons with a Dementia through Radical Reflection and Participation. Thesis for Doctorate in Philosophy (PhD), University of Manchester, Manchester.

Dewing, J. (2008a). Process consent and research with older persons living with dementia. *Association of Research Ethics Journal*, 4(2), 59–64.

Dewing, J. (2008b). Becoming and Being Active Learners and Creating Active Learning Workplaces: The Value of Active Learning. In K. Manley, B. McCormack & V. Wilson (Eds), *International Practice Development in Nursing and Healthcare* (Chapter 15, pp. 273–294). Oxford: Blackwell.

Dewing, J. (2008c). Personhood and dementia: revisiting Tom Kitwood's ideas. *International Journal of Older People Nursing*, 3, 3–13.

Dillon, M.C. (1988). *Merleau-Ponty's Ontology*, 2nd Edn. Illinois: Northwestern University Press.

Donabedian, A. (1982). *Explorations in Quality Assessment and Monitoring Volume II: The Criteria and Standards of Quality*. Michigan: Health Administration Press.

Down, J. (2004). From Conception to Delivery – a Journey towards a Trust-wide Strategy to Develop a Culture of Patient-Centredness. In B. McCormack, K. Manley & R. Garbett (Eds), *Practice Development in Nursing* (pp. 267–287). Oxford: Blackwell.

Downie, R.S. & Calman, K.C. (1994). *Healthy Respect: Ethics in Health Care*. Oxford: Oxford University Press.

Dreyfus, H.L. & Dreyfus, S.E. (1986). *Mind over Machine: The Power of Human Intuition and Expertise in the Era of the Computer*. New York: The Free Press.

Duffield, C., Roche, M., O'Brien-Pallas, L., Diers, D., Aisbett, C., King, M., Aisbett, K. & Hall, J. (2007). *Glueing it Together: Nurses, their Work Environment and Patient Safety*. Sydney: Centre for Health Services Management, University of Technology.

Dworkin, G. (1989). The Concept of Autonomy. In J. Christman (Ed.), *The Inner Citadel: Essays on Individual Autonomy*. Oxford: Oxford University Press.

Dworkin, G. (1991). *The Theory and Practice of Autonomy*. Cambridge: Cambridge University Press.

Edwards, C. & Staniszewska, S. (2000). Accessing the user's perspective. *Health and Social Care in the Community*, 8(6), 417–424.

Edwards, C., Staniszweska, S. & Crichton, N. (2004). Investigation of the ways in which patients' reports of their satisfaction with healthcare are constructed. *Sociology of Health & Illness*, 26(2), 159–183.

Edwards, S.D. (2001). *Philosophy of Nursing: An Introduction*. Basingstoke, Hampshire: Palgrave.

Elliott, J. (2008). "Dance Mirrors": Embodying, Actualizing and Operationalizing a Dance Experience in a Healthcare Context. Unpublished Doctoral Thesis, University of Ulster, Jordanstown, Northern Ireland.

Ellis, S. (1999). The patient-centred care model: holistic/multidisciplinary/reflective. *British Journal of Nursing*, 8(5), 296–301.

Entwistle, V. & Watt, I. (2006). Patient involvement in treatment decision-making: the case for a broader conceptual framework. *Patient Education and Counselling*, 63, 268–278.

Entwistle, V.A., Watt, I.S., Gilhooly, K., Bugge, C., Haites, N. & Walker, A.E. (2004). Assessing patients' participation and quality of decision-making: insights from a study of routine practice in diverse settings. *Patient Education and Counselling*, 55, 105–113.

Ericson, I., Hellstrom, I., Lundh, U. & Nolan, M. (2001). What constitutes good care for people with dementia? *British Journal of Nursing*, 10(11), 710–714.

Estabrooks, C.A., Midodzi, W.K., Cummings, G.G., Ricker, K.L. & Giovannetti, P. (2005). The impact of hospital nursing characteristics on 30-day mortality. *Nursing Research*, 54(2), 74–84.

European Commission (2005). Improving the mental health of the population: towards a strategy on mental health for the European Union. (Green Paper) COM (2005)484. Brussels: EU Health and Consumer Protection Directorate-General.

Evans, L.K. (1996). Knowing the patient: the route to individualised care. *Journal of Gerontological Nursing*, 22(3), 15–19.

Fanon, F. (1967). *The Wretched of the Earth*. London: Penguin.

Farrell, G.A. (1999). Aggression in clinical settings: nurses' views – a follow-up study. *Journal of Advanced Nursing*, 29(3), 532–541.

Farrell, G.A. (2001). From tall poppies to squashed weeds: why don't nurses pull together more? *Journal of Advanced Nursing*, 35(1), 26–33.

Fawcett, J. (1995). *Analysis and Evaluation of Conceptual Models of Nursing*, 3rd Edn. Philadelphia: F.A. Davis Company.

Fay, B. (1987). *Critical Social Science: Liberation and Its Limits*. Cambridge: Polity Press.

Finfgeld-Connett, D. (2008). Meta-synthesis of caring in nursing. *Journal of Clinical Nursing*, 17, 196–204.

Finn, C.P. (2001). Autonomy: an important component of nurses' job satisfaction. *International Journal of Nursing Studies*, 38(3), 349–357.

Ford, J.S. (1990). Caring encounters. *Scandinavian Journal of Caring Sciences*, 4, 157–162.

Ford, P. & McCormack, B. (2000). Future directions for gerontology: a nursing perspective. *Nurse Education Today*, 20(5), 389–394.

Fosbinder, D. (1994). Patient perceptions of nursing care: an emerging theory of interpersonal competence. *Journal of Advanced Nursing*, 20, 1085–1093.

Foucault, M. (1982). The subject and power. *Critical Inquiry*, 8(Summer), 777–795.

Frampton, S.B. (2003). *Putting Patients First: Designing and Practicing Patient-Centered Care*. San Francisco, CA: John Wiley and Sons.

Frankfurt, H.G. (1989). Freedom of the Will and the Concept of a Person. In J. Christman (Ed.), *The Inner Citadel: Essays on Individual Autonomy*. Oxford: Oxford University Press.

Freshwater, D. (2000). Crosscurrents: against cultural narration in nursing. *Journal of Advanced Nursing*, 32(2), 481–484.

Fry, S.T. (1989). Towards a theory of nursing ethics. *Advances in Nursing Science*, 11, 9–22.

Fulford, K.W.M., Ersser, S. & Hope, T. (1996). *Essential Practice in Patient-Centred Care*. Oxford: Blackwell Science.

Gadamer, H.G. (1993). *Truth and Method*. London: Sheed & Ward.

Gadow, S. (1980). Existential Advocacy: Philosophical Foundations of Nursing. In S.F. Spicker & S. Gadow (Eds), *Nursing: Images and Ideals – Opening Dialogue with the Humanities.* New York: Springer.

Gadow, S. (1990). Existential Advocacy: Philosophical Foundations of Nursing. In T. Pence & J. Cantrell (Eds) *Ethics in Nursing: An Anthology.* New York: National League for Nursing.

Gadow, S.A. (1985). Nurse and Patient: The Caring Relationship. In A.H. Bishop & J.R. Scudder (Eds), *Caring, Curing and Coping* (pp. 31–43). Alabama: The University of Alabama Press.

Gamez, G.G. (2009). The nurse–patient relationship as a caring relationship. *Nursing Science Quarterly,* 22(2), 126–127.

Garbett, R. & McCormack, B. (2002). A concept analysis of practice development. *NT Research,* 7(2), 87–100.

Garbett, R., Hardy, S., Manley, K., Titchen, A. & McCormack, B. (2007). Developing a qualitative approach to 360-degree feedback to aid understanding and development of clinical expertise. *Journal of Nursing Management,* 15(3), 342–347.

Gardner, H. (1993). *Frames of Mind.* New York: Basic Books.

Gaut, D.A. (1983). Development of a theoretically adequate description of caring. *Western Journal of Nursing Research,* 5, 313–324.

Gaylin, W. (1979). *Caring.* New York: Avon Books.

Genevay, B. & Katz, R.S. (1990). *Countertransference and Older Clients.* London: Sage.

Gilligan, C. (1982). *In a Different Voice: Psychological Theory and Women's Development.* Cambridge Massachusetts & London: Harvard University Press.

Gleason-Scott, J., Sochalski, J. & Aiken, L. (1999). Review of magnet hospitals research. *Journal of Nursing Administration,* 29(1), 9–19.

Goffman, E. (1961). *On the Characteristics of Total Institutions. First Essay in Asylums.* Harmondsworth: Penguin.

Goldsmith, M. (1996). *Hearing the Voices of People with Dementia: Opportunities and Obstacles.* London: Jessica Kingsley Publishers.

Goleman, D. (1996). *Emotional Intelligence – Why It Can Matter More Than IQ.* London: Bloomsbury.

Goleman, D. (1999). *Working with Emotional Intelligence.* London: Bloomsbury.

Gould, D. (1990). Empathy: a review of the literature with suggestions for an alternative research strategy. *Journal of Advanced Nursing,* 15(11), 1167–1174.

Griffin, A.P. (1983). A philosophical analysis of caring in nursing. *Journal of Advanced Nursing,* 8, 289–295.

Guba, E.G. & Lincoln, Y.S. (1989). *Fourth Generation Evaluation.* Newbury Park: Sage.

Gunnarsdóttir, S.G., Clarke, S.P., Rafferty, A.M. & Nutbeam, D. (2009). Front-line management, staffing and nurse-doctor relationships as predictors of nurse and patient outcomes. A survey of Icelandic hospital nurses. *International Journal of Nursing Studies,* 46(7), 920–927.

Hale, C. (1986). Measuring job satisfaction. *Nursing Times,* 82(5), 43–46.

Hallsdorsdottir, S. & Hamrin, E. (1997). Caring and uncaring encounters within nursing and healthcare from the cancer patients perspective. *Cancer Nursing,* 20(2), 120–128.

Hannemann, B.T. (2006). Creativity with dementia patients: can creativity and art stimulate dementia patients positively. *Gerontology,* 52(1), 59–65.

Hardy, S., Titchen, A., Manley, K. & McCormack, B. (2006). Re-defining nursing expertise in the United Kingdom. *Nursing Science Quarterly*, 19(3), 260–264.

Hardy, S., Manley, K., Titchen, A. & McCormack, B. (Eds) (2009). *Revealing Nursing Expertise through Practitioner Enquiry*. Oxford: Wiley-Blackwell Publishing.

Harrison, L.L. (1990). Guest editorial: maintaining the ethic of caring in nursing. *Journal of Advanced Nursing*, 15, 125–127.

Harvey, G., Loftus-Hills, A., Rycroft-Malone, J., Titchen, A., Kitson, A., McCormack, B. & Seers, K. (2002). Getting evidence into practice: the role and function of facilitation. *Journal of Advanced Nursing*, 37(6), 577–588.

Hayes, L.J., O'Brien-Pallas, L., Duffield, C., Shamian, J., Buchan, J., Hughes, F., Spence Laschinger, H.K., North, N. & Stone, P.W. (2006). Nurse turnover: a literature review. *International Journal of Nursing Studies*, 43, 237–263.

Heidegger, M. (1962). *Being and Time (Reprinted Version 1980)*. Oxford: Basil Blackwell.

Heidegger, M. (1990). *Being and Time*. Oxford: Basil Blackwell.

Heron, J. (1989). *The Facilitators' Handbook*. London: Kogan Page.

Hoeffer, B., Talerico, K.A., Raisin, J., Mitchell, M., Stewart, B.J., McKenzie, D., Barrick, A.L., Rader, J. & Sloane, P.D. (2006). Assisting cognitively impaired nursing home residents with bathing: effects of two bathing interventions on caregiving. *The Gerontologist*, 46(4), 524–532.

Hoff, T., Pohl, H. & Bartfield, J. (2004). Creating a learning environment to produce competent residents: the roles of culture and context. *Academic Medicine*, 6, 532–540.

Holden, R.J. (1990). Empathy: the art of emotional knowing in holistic nursing care. *Holistic Nursing Practice*, 5(1), 70–79.

Hope, K.W. & Waterman, H. (2004). 'Finding the person the disease has' – the case for multisensory environments. *Journal of Psychiatric and Mental Health Nursing*, 11, 554–561.

Horton, K., Tschudin, V. & Forget, A. (2007). The value of nursing: a literature review. *Nursing Ethics*, 14(6), 716–740.

Hospice Friendly Hospitals Programme (2008). *Design and Dignity Guidelines for Physical Environments of Hospitals Supporting End-of-Life Care*. The Irish Hospice Foundation, Dublin, Ireland www.hospicefriendlyhospitals.net

Hsu, M.-Y. & McCormack, B. (2006). *Using Older Peoples' Stories to Inform Service Development*. Final Report to the BUPA Foundation. April 2006, University of Ulster http://www.science.ulster.ac.uk/inr/pdf/finalreport_bupa.pdf (accessed April 2009).

Hussain, F. & Raczka, R. (1997). Life story work for people with learning disabilities. *British Journal of Learning Disabilities*, 25(2), 73–76.

Jacono, B.J. (1993). Caring is loving. *Journal of Advanced in Nursing*, 18, 192–194.

James, N. (1992). Care = organisation + physical labour + emotional labour. *Sociology of Health and Illness*, 14(4), 489–509.

Jameton, A. (1984). *Nursing Practice: The Ethical Issues*. Englewood Cliffs, New Jersey: Prentice-Hall.

Jecker, N.S. & Self, D.J. (1991). Separating care and cure: an analysis of historical and contemporary images of nursing and medicine. *The Journal of Medicine and Philosophy*, 16, 285–306.

Johns, C. (1994). *The Burford NDU Model – Caring in Practice*. Oxford: Blackwell.

Johns, C. (1998). Opening the Doors of Perception. In C. Johns & D. Freshwater (Eds), *Transforming Nursing through Reflective Practice*. Oxford: Blackwell Science.

Johns, C. (1999). Reflection as empowerment. *Nursing Inquiry*, 6(4), 241–249.

Johns, C. (2005). Appreciating (guided) reflection as a process of self-inquiry and transformation toward realizing desirable practice. *International Journal of Human Caring*, 9(2), 139.

Johns, C.C. (1991). *Becoming a Primary Nurse*. Burford, Oxon: BNDU Publications.

Johns, C.C. (1995). Achieving Effective Work as Professional Activity. In J.E. Schober & S.M. Hinchliff (Eds), *Towards Advanced Practice: Key Concepts for Health Care*. London: Arnold.

Johnson, M. (1991). The Meaning of Old Age. In S.J. Redfern (Ed.), *Nursing Elderly People*. Edinburgh: Churchill Livingstone.

Kane, R., Lun, T., Cutler, L., Degenholtz, H. & Tzy-Chyi, Y. (2007). Resident outcomes in small-house nursing homes: a longitudinal evaluation of the Initial Green House Program. *American Geriatrics Society*, 55, 832–839.

Kaye, B.L. & Jordan-Evans, S. (2005). *Love 'Em or Lose 'Em: Getting Good People to Stay*. San Francisco: Berrett-Koehler Publishers.

Keane, S.M., Chastain, B. & Rudisill, K. (1987). Caring: nurse–patient perceptions. *Rehabilitation Nursing*, 12, 182–184.

Kelly, L.S. (1988). The ethic of caring: has it been discarded? *Nursing Outlook*, 36, 17.

Kenyon, G. Clark, P. & deVries, B. (2001). *Narrative Gerontology: Theory, Research and Practice*. New York: Springer Publishing Company.

Kim, H.S. (1998). Critical reflective inquiry for knowledge development in nursing practice. *Journal of Advanced Nursing*, 29(5), 1205–1212.

Kitson, A., Harvey, G. & McCormack, B. (1998). Approaches to implementing research in practice. *Quality in Health Care*, 7(3), 149–159.

Kitson, A.L. (1987). A comparative analysis of lay caring and professional (nursing) care relationships. *International Journal of Nursing Studies*, 24(2), 155–165.

Kitwood, T. (1997). *Dementia Reconsidered: The Person Comes First*. Milton Keynes: Open University Press.

Kitwood, T. & Bredin, K. (1992). A new approach to the evaluation of dementia care. *Journal of Advances in Health and Nursing Care*, 1(5), 41–60.

Komorita, N.I., Doehring, K.M. & Hirchert, P.W. (1991). Perceptions of caring by nurse educators. *Journal of Nursing Education*, 30, 23–29.

Kouzes, J. & Posner, B. (2002a). *The Leadership Challenge*, 3rd Edn. San Francisco, CA: Jossey-Bass.

Kouzes, J.M. & Posner, B.Z. (2002b). The Leadership Practices Inventory: Theory and Evidence behind the Five Practices of Exemplary Leaders. http://media.wiley.com/assets/463/74/lc_jb_appendix.pdf (accessed April 2009).

Kouzes, J.M. & Posner, B.Z. (2003). *The Five Practices of Exemplary Leadership*. San Francisco, CA: Pfeiffer.

Kouzes, J.M. & Posner, B.Z. (2007). *The Leadership Challenge*, 4th Edn. San Francisco: Jossey-Bass.

Kramer, M. & Hafner, L.P. (1989). Shared values: impact on staff nurse job satisfaction and perceived productivity. *Nursing Research*, 38(3), 172–177.

Large, S., Macleod, A., Cunningham, G. & Kitson, A. (2005). A Multiple Case Study Evaluation of the RCN Clinical Leadership Programme in England. London: Royal College of Nursing Institute. http://www.rcn .org.uk/__data/assets/pdf_file/0010/78643/002502.pdf

Larson, P.J. (1981). Oncology Patients and Professional Nurses' Perception of Important Caring Behaviors. PhD Thesis, University of California, San Francisco.

Laschinger, H.K.S., Finegan, J., Shamian, J. & Casier, S. (2000). Organisational trust and empowerment in restructured healthcare settings: effects on staff nurse commitment. *Journal of Nursing Administration*, 30(9), 413–425.

Laschinger, H.K.S., Finegan, J. & Shamian, J. (2001). Promoting nurses' health: effect of empowerment on job strain and work satisfaction. *Nursing Economics*, 19(2), 42–52.

Laschinger, H.K.S., Almost, J. & Tuer-Hodes, D. (2003). Workplace empowerment and magnet hospital characteristics – making the link. *Journal of Nursing Administration*, 33(7–8), 410–422.

Laverack, G. (2005). *Public Health: Power and Professional Practice*. London: Palgrave Macmillan.

Lea, A. & Watson, R. (1995). Different conceptions of caring: mental health and general nurses. *Journal of Psychiatric and Mental Health Nursing*, 2, 184.

Lea, A. & Watson, R. (1999). Perceptions of caring among nurses: the relationship to clinical areas. *Journal of Clinical Nursing*, 8(5), 617.

Leddy, S. & Pepper, J.M. (1993). *Conceptual Bases of Professional Nursing*. Philadelphia: JB Lippincott.

Leininger, M.M. (1981). Some Philosophic, Historical, and Taxonomic Aspects of Nursing and Caring in American Culture. In M.M. Leininger (Ed.), *Caring: An Essential Human Need* (pp. 133–143). Detroit: Wayne State University Press.

Leplege, A., Gzil, F., Cammelli, M., Lefeve, C., Pachoud, B. & Ville, I. (2007). Person-centredness: conceptual and historical perspectives. *Disability and Rehabilitation*, 29(20–21), 1555–1565.

Lewis, C.K. & Matthews, J.H. (1998). Magnet program designates exceptional nursing sources. *American Journal of Nursing*, 98(12), 51–52.

Lin, Y. & Chiou, C. (2003). Concept analysis of caring. *Journal of Nursing*, 50(6), 74–78.

Loane, P.D., HOeffer, B., Mtchell, M., Mcenzie, D.A., Barrick, A.L., Radar, J., Stewart, B.J., Talerico, K.A., Rasin, J.H., Zink, R.C. & Koch, G.G. (2004). Effect of person-centred showering and the towel bath on bathing-associated aggression, agitation, and discomfort in nursing home residents with dementia: a randomized, controlled trial. *Journal of the American Geriatric Society*, 52, 1795–1804.

Longo, J. & Sherman, R. (2007). Leveling horizontal violence. *Nursing Management*, 38(3), 34–37, 50–51.

Lowson, K., Beale, S., Kelly, J. & Hadfield, M. (2006). *Evaluation of Enhancing the Healing Environment Programme*. Final Report for the Department of Health (NHS Estates), York Health Economics Consortium, University of York, York, England.

Luckhurst, M. & Ray, M. (1999). Person-centred standards of care. *Elderly Care*, 11(6), 29–31.

Luft, J. (1984). *Group Processes – An Introduction to Group Dynamics.* California: Mayfield.

Maben, J. & Griffiths, P. (2008). *Nurses in Society: Starting the Debate.* London: National Nursing Research Unit.

MacIntyre, A. (1992). *After Virtue – A Study in Moral Theory.* London: Duckworth.

Malinski, V.M. (2009). Intentionality, consciousness and creating community. *Nursing Science Quarterly*, 22(1), 13–14.

Mangold, A.M. (1991). Senior nursing students' and professional nurses' perceptions of effective caring behaviors: a comparative study. *Journal of Nursing Education*, 30, 137–139.

Manley, K. (1996). Job satisfaction in intensive care among nurses practicing primary nursing and a comparison with those practicing total patient care. *Nursing in Critical Care*, 1(1), 31–41.

Manley, K. (2000a). Organisational culture and consultant nurse outcomes: part 1 organisational culture. *Nursing Standard*, 14, 34–38.

Manley, K. (2000b). Organisational culture and consultant nurse outcomes: part 2 consultant nurse outcomes. *Nursing Standard*, 14, 34–39.

Manley, K. (2001). Consultant Nurse: Concept, Processes, Outcomes. Unpublished PhD, University of Manchester/RCN, London.

Manley, K. (2004). Transformational Culture: A Culture of Effectiveness. In B. McCormack, K. Manley & R. Garbett (Eds), *Practice Development in Nursing* (pp. 51–82). Oxford: Blackwell Publishing.

Manley, K. & McCormack, B. (1997). *Exploring Expert Practice.* London: RCN.

Manley, K. & McCormack, B. (2004). Practice Development: Purpose, Methodology, Facilitation and Evaluation. In B. McCormack, K. Manley & R. Garbett (Eds), *Practice Development in Nursing.* Oxford: Blackwell Publishing.

Manley, K., Hardy, S., Titchen, A., Garbett, A. & McCormack, B. (2005). *Research Reports: Changing Patients' Worlds through Nursing Practice Expertise: Exploring Nursing Practice Experience through Emancipator Action Research and Fourth Generation Evaluation.* London: Royal College of Nursing.

Manley, K., McCormack, B. & Wilson, V. (2008). Introduction. In K. Manley, B. McCormack & V. Wilson (Eds), *Practice Development in Nursing: International Perspectives* (pp. 1–16). Oxford: Blackwell Publishing.

Manley, K., Titchen, A. & Hardy, S. (2009). From Artistry in Practice to Expertise in Developing Person-Centred Systems: A Clinical Career Framework. In S. Hardy, A. Titchen, B. McCormack & K. Manley (Eds), *Revealing Nursing Expertise through Practitioner Inquiry* (pp. 3–30). Oxford: Wiley-Blackwell.

Manojlovich, M. & Laschinger, H. (2007). The nursing worklife model: extending and refining a new theory. *Journal of Nursing Management*, 15, 256–263.

Manthey, M. (2002). *The Practice of Primary Nursing.* Indianapolis, IN: Creative Healthcare.

Marcel, G. (1981). *The Philosophy of Existence (Edited and translated by R.R. Grabon).* Philadelphia: University of Pennsylvania Press.

Martin, G.W. & Younger, D. (2001). Person-centred care for people with dementia: a quality audit approach. *Journal of Psychiatric and Mental Health Nursing*, 8(5), 443–448.

Masterson, A. (2007). Community matrons: the value of knowing self (part two). *Nursing Older People*, 5, 29–31.

Mayer, D.K. (1987). Oncology nurses' versus cancer patients' perceptions of nurse caring behaviors: a replication study. *Oncology Nurses' Forum*, 14, 48–52.

Mayeroff, M. (1971). *On Caring*. London: Harper Row.

McCabe, C. (2004). Nurse–patient communication: an exploration of patients experiences. *Journal of Clinical Nursing*, 13, 41–49.

McCance, T.V. (1999). An Exploration of the Experience of Caring in Nursing: A Hermeneutic Approach. Unpublished DPhil Thesis, University of Ulster, Northern Ireland.

McCance, T.V. (2003). Caring in nursing practice: the development of a conceptual framework. *Research and Theory for Nursing Practice: An International Journal*, 17(2), 101–116.

McCance, T.V., McKenna, H.P. & Boore, J.R.P. (1997). Caring: dealing with a difficult concept. *International Journal of Nursing Studies*, 34, 241–248.

McCance, T.V., McKenna, H.P. & Boore, J.R.P. (1999). Caring: theoretical perspectives of relevance to nursing. *Journal of Advanced Nursing*, 30, 1388–1395.

McCance, T.V., McKenna, H.P. & Boore, J.R.P. (2001). Exploring caring using narrative methodology: an analysis of the approach. *Journal of Advanced Nursing*, 33, 350–356.

McCance, T., Slater, P. & McCormack, B. (2008). Using the caring dimensions inventory (CDI) as an indicator of person-centred nursing. *Journal of Clinical Nursing*, 18, 409–417.

McCance, T., Gribben, B., McCormack, B. & Mitchell, E. (2010). *Improving the patient experience by exploring person-centred care in practice*. Final Programme Report, Belfast Health & Social Care Trust, Belfast.

McCarthy, B. (2006). Translating person-centred care: a case study of preceptor nurses and their teaching practices in acute care areas. *Journal of Clinical Nursing*, 15(5), 629–638.

McClure, M., Poulin, M., Sovie, M. & Wandelt, M. (1983). *Magnet Hospitals: Attraction and Retention of Professional Nurses*. Kansas City: American Academy of Nursing Taskforce on Nursing Practice in Hospitals.

McCormack, B. (1992). 'Intuition': concept analysis and application to curriculum development. Part 1: concept analysis. *Journal of Clinical Nursing*, 1, 339–344.

McCormack, B. (2001a). Autonomy and the relationship between nurses and older people. *Ageing and Society*, 21, 417–446.

McCormack, B. (2001b). *Negotiating Partnerships with Older People: A Person-Centred Approach*. Basingstoke: Ashgate.

McCormack, B. (2002). The person of the voice: narrative identities in informed consent. *Nursing Philosophy*, 3, 114–119, Blackwell Science Ltd.

McCormack, B. (2003). A conceptual framework for person-centred practice with older people. *International Journal of Nursing Practice*, 9, 202–209.

McCormack, B. (2004). Person-centredness in gerontological nursing: an overview of the literature. *Journal of Clinical Nursing*, 13(3A), 31–38.

McCormack, B. (2009). Practitioner Research. In S. Hardy, K. Manley, A. Titchen & B. McCormack (Eds), *Expertise in Nursing Practice*. Oxford: Blackwell Publishing.

McCormack, B. & McCance, T.V. (2006). Developing a conceptual framework for person-centred nursing. *Journal of Advanced Nursing*, 56(5), 472–479.

McCormack, B. & Titchen, A. (2006). Critical creativity: melding, exploding, blending. *Educational Action Research*, 14(2), 239–266.

McCormack, B., Kitson, A., Harvey, G., Rycroft-Malone, J., Titchen, A. & Seers, K. (2002). Getting evidence into practice: the meaning of 'context'. *Journal of Advanced Nursing*, 38(1), 94–104.

McCormack, B., Devlin, M. & McIlrath, C. (2004). *REACH Pilot 1a Evaluation*. Belfast: Royal Hospitals Trust and Royal College of Nursing.

McCormack, B., Wright, J., Dewer, B., Harvey, G. & Ballintine, K. (2007). A realist synthesis of evidence relating to practice development: interviews and synthesis of data. *Practice Development in Health Care*, 6(1), 56–75.

McCormack, B., Manley, K. & Walsh, K. (2008a). Person-Centred Systems and Processes. In K. Manley, B. McCormack & V. Wilson (Eds), *International Practice Development in Nursing and Healthcare* (pp. 17–41). Oxford: Blackwell.

McCormack, B., McCance, T., Slater, P., McCormick, J., McArdle, C. & Dewing, J. (2008b). Person-Centred Outcomes and Cultural Change. In K. Manley, B. McCormack & V. Wilson (Eds), *International Practice Development in Nursing and Healthcare* (pp. 189–214). Oxford: Blackwell.

McCormack, B., Henderson, E., Wilson, V. & Wright, J. (2009a). The workplace culture critical analysis tool. *Practice Development in Healthcare*, 8(1), 28–43.

McCormack, B., McCarthy, G., Wright, J., Slater, P. & Coffey, A. (2009b). Development and testing of the context assessment index. *Worldviews on Evidence Based Nursing*, 6(1), 27–35.

McCormack, B., Dewing, J., Breslin, L., Coyne-Nevin, A., Kennedy, K., Manning, M., Peelo-Kilroe, L. & Tobin, C. (2009c). *Practice Development: Realising active learning for sustainable change, Contemporary Nurse*, 32(1–2): 92–104.

McFarlane, J.K. (1976). A charter for caring. *Journal of Advanced Nursing*, 1, 187–196.

McGregor, M. (2003). Cost-utility analysis: use QALYs only with great caution. *Journal of the Canadian Medical Association*, 168(4), 433–434.

Mckenna, B., Smith, N.A., Poole, S.J. & Coverdale, J.H. (2002). Horizontal violence: experiences of registered nurses in their first year of practice. *Journal of Advanced Nursing*, 42(1), 90–96.

McMurray, J. (1995). *The Self as Agent: The Form of the Personal*. London: Faber and Faber.

McNeese-Smith, D. (1993). Leadership behavior and employee effectiveness. *Nursing Management*, 24(5), 38–39.

McNeese-Smith, D. (1995). Job satisfaction, productivity, and organizational commitment. The result of leadership. *Journal of Nursing Administration*, 25(9), 17–26.

McQueen, A. (2000). Nurse–patient relationships and partnership in hospital care. *Journal of Clinical Nursing*, 9, 723–731.

Medvene, L., Grosch, K. & Swink, N. (2006). Interpersonal complexity: a cognitive component of person-centred care. *Gerontologist*, 46(2), 220–226.

Merleau-Ponty, M. (1962). *The Phenomenology of Perception (Translated by C. Smith)*. London: Routledge and Kegan Paul.

Merleau-Ponty, M. (1989). *Phenomenology of Perception (Translation by C. Smith with revisions by F. Williams and D. Gurriere)*. London: Routledge.

Meyer, J. & Sturdy, D. (2004). Exploring the future of gerontological nursing outcomes. *International Journal of Older People Nursing*, 13(6b), 128–134.

Meyers, D.T. (1989). *Self, Society and Personal Choice*. New York: Columbia University Press.

Mezirow, J. (1981). A critical theory of adult learning and education. *Adult Education Quarterly*, 32(1), 3–24.

Mezirow, J. (1991). *Fostering Critical Reflection in Adulthood*. San Francisco: Jossey-Bass.

Mitchell, P.H., Ferketich, S. & Jennings, B.M. (1998). Quality health outcomes model. American Academy of Nursing Expert Panel on Quality Health Care. *Image Journal of Nursing Scholarship*, 30(1), 43–46.

Molina, F. (1962). *Existentialism as Philosophy*. New Jersey: Prentice-Hall Inc.

Montalvo, I. (2007). The National Database of Nursing Quality Indicators (NDNQI®). *OJIN: The Online Journal of Issues in Nursing*, 12(3), Manuscript 2. www.nursingworld.org/MainMenuCategories/ANAMarketplace/ANAPeriodicals/OJIN/TableofContents/Volume122007/No3Sept07/NursingQualityIndicators.aspx.

Morrison, P. (1991). The caring attitude in nursing practice: a repertory grid study of trained nurses' perceptions. *Nurse Education Today*, 11, 3–12.

Morse, J., Bottorff, J., Anderson, G., O'Brien, B. & Solberg, S. (2006). Beyond empathy: expanding expressions of caring. *Journal of Advanced Nursing*, 53(1), 75–90.

Morse, J.M., Bottorff, J., Neander, W. & Solberg, S. (1991). Comparative analysis of conceptualizations and theories of caring. *Journal of Nursing Scholarship*, 23(2), 119–126.

Morse, J.M., Bottorff, J.L., Anderson, G., O'Brien, B. & Solberg, S. (1992). Beyond empathy: expanding expressions of caring. *Journal of Advanced Nursing*, 17, 809–821.

National Institute for Clinical Excellence (2004). *Improving Supportive and Palliative Care for Adults with Cancer*. London: NICE.

National Nursing Research Unit (2008). *State of the Art Metrics for Nursing: A Rapid Appraisal*. London: Kings College London.

Neuman, B. (1996). The Neuman systems model in research and practice. *Nursing Science Quarterly*, 9, 67–70.

Newman, K., Maylor, U. & Chansarkar, B. (2001). The nurse retention, quality of care and patient satisfaction chain. *International Journal of Health Care Quality Assurance*, 14(2), 57–68.

Niebhur, H.R. (1963). *The Responsible Self: An Essay in Christian Moral Philosophy*. New York: Harper & Row.

Nieva, V.F. & Sorra, J. (2003). Safety culture assessment: a tool for improving patient safety in healthcare organizations. *Quality and Safety in Health Care*, 12, 17–23.

Nolan, M. (2001). Successful ageing: keeping the 'person' in person-centred care. *British Journal of Nursing*, 10(7), 450–454.

Nolan, M., Davies, S. & Grant, G. (2001). *Working with Older People and Their Families: Key Issues in Policy and Practice*. Buckingham: Open University Press.

Nolan, M., Davies, S., Brown, J., Keady, J. & Nolan, J. (2004). Beyond 'person-centred' care: a new vision for gerontological nursing. *International Journal of Older People Nursing [in association with the Journal of Clinical Nursing]*, 13(3a), 45–53.

Nolan, T.W. (2007). *Execution of Strategic Improvement Initiatives to Produce System-Level Results*. IHI Innovation Series white paper. Cambridge, MA: Institute for Healthcare Improvement. (Available on www.IHI.org).

Northern Ireland Practice and Education Council (2006). *Competency Profile. Foundation Paper*. Belfast: NIPEC.

Nursing and Midwifery Council (2009). *Guidance for the Care of Older People*. London: NMC.

O'Brien-Pallas, L., Griffin, P., Shamian, J., Buchan, J., Duffield, C., Hughes, F., Spence Laschinger, H.K., North, N. & Stone, P.W. (2008). The impact of nurse turnover on patient, nurse, and system outcomes: a pilot study and focus for a multicentre international study. *Policy, Politics and Nursing Practice*, 7(3), 169–179.

Oermann, M.H. & Bizek, K.S. (1994). Job satisfaction among critical care preceptors. *Critical Care Nursing*, 14, 3–6.

Packer, T. (2003). Turning Rhetoric into Reality: Person-Centred Approaches for Community Mental Health Nursing. In J. Keady, C. Clarke & T. Adams (Eds), *Community Mental Health Nursing and Dementia Care* (pp. 104–119). Maidenhead: Open University Press.

Parley, F.F. (2001). Person-centred outcomes – are outcomes improved where a person-centred care model is used? *Journal of Learning Disabilities*, 5(4), 299–308.

Paterson, J.G. & Zderad, L.T. (1988). *Humanistic Nursing*, 2nd Edn. New York: National League for Nursing.

Paton, H.J. (1964). *Groundwork of the Metaphysics of Morals*. New York: Harper & Row.

Pawson, R. & Tilley, N. (1997). *Realistic Evaluation*. London: Sage.

Peplau, H.E. (1952). *Interpersonal Relations in Nursing*. Philadelphia: Putnam's Sons.

Phillips, C. & Thompson, G. (2009). *What is a QALY*. Hayward Medical Communications http://www.evidence-based-medicine.co.uk/ebmfiles/WhatisaQALY.pdf (accessed April 2009).

Pike, A.W. (1990). On the nature and place of empathy in clinical nursing practice. *Journal of Professional Nursing*, 6(4), 235–241.

Plas, J. & Lewis, S. (2001). *Person-Centered Leadership for Nonprofit Organisations*. Thousand oaks: Sage Publications.

Platzer, H., Blake, D. & Ashford, D. (2000). An evaluation of process and outcomes from learning through reflective practice groups on a post-registration nursing course. *Journal of Advanced Nursing*, 31(3), 689–695.

Plsek, P.E. (2001). Redesigning Health Care with Insights from the Science of Complex Adaptive Systems. In *Crossing the Chasm: A New Health System for the 21st Century*. Washington: National Academy Press.

Plsek, P.E. & Greenhalgh, T. (2001). The challenge of complexity in health care. *British Medical Journal*, 323, 625–628.

Policy+ (2008). Can you measure nursing? *Policy+* – Policy plus evidence, issues and opinions in healthcare, Issue 12 (October 2008) National Nursing Research Unit, King's College, London. http://www.kcl.ac.uk/content/1/c6/02/56/58/PolicyIssue12.pdf (accessed April 2009).

Pope, R., Graham, L. & Patel, S. (2001). Woman-centred care. *International Journal of Nursing Studies*, 38, 227–238.

Porter-O'Grady, T. (2003). A different age for leadership, part 2: new rules, new roles. *Journal of Nursing Administration*, 33(3), 173–178.

Post, S. (2006). Respectare: Moral Respect for the Lives of the Deeply Forgetful. In J.C. Hughes, S.J. Louw & S.R. Sabat (Eds), *Dementia: Mind, Meaning and the Person*. Oxford: Oxford University Press.

Prieto, L. & Sacristán, J. (2003). Problems and solutions in calculating quality-adjusted life years (QALYs). *Health and Quality of Life Outcomes*. Issue 1 http://www.ncbi.nlm.nih.gov/pmc/articles/PMC317370/pdf/1477-7525-1-80.pdf.

Rafferty, A.M., Clarke, S.P., Coles, J., Ball, J., James, P., McKee, M. & Aiken, L.H. (2007). Outcomes of variation in hospital nurse staffing in English hospitals: cross-sectional analysis of survey data and discharge records. *International Nursing of Nursing Studies*, 44, 175–182.

Rawls, J. (1992). *A Theory of Justice*. Oxford: Oxford University Press.

Ray, M.A. (1981). A Philosophical Analysis of Caring within Nursing. In M.M. Leininger (Ed.), *Caring: An Essential Human Need* (pp. 25–36). Detroit: Wayne State University Press.

Ray, M.A. (1987). Technological caring: a new model for critical care. *Dimensions of Critical Care Nursing*, 6, 166–173.

Redfern, S., Christian, S. & Norman, I. (2003). Evaluating change in health care practice: lessons from three studies. *Journal of Evaluation in Clinical Practice*, 9, 239–249.

Reed, J. (2007). *Appreciative Inquiry: Research for Change*. London: Sage.

Reiman, D.J. (1986). Noncaring and caring in the clinical setting: patients' descriptions. *Topics of Clinical Nursing*, 8, 30–36.

Roach, S. (1984). *Caring: The Human Mode of Being*. Toronto: University of Toronto.

Robbins, D.A. (1996). *Ethical and Legal Issues in Home Health and Long-Term Care: Challenges and Solutions*. Maryland: Aspen Publishers, Inc.

Robertson, J., Hatton, C., Emerson, E., Elliott, J., McIntosh, B., Swift, P., Krinjen-Kemp, E., Towers, C., Romeo, R., Knapp, M., Sanderson, H., Routledge, M., Oakes, P. & Joyce, T. (2007). Reported barriers to the implementation of person-centred planning for people with intellectual disabilities in the UK. *Journal of Applied Research in Intellectual Disabilities*, 20(4), 297–307.

Rogers, C. (1961). *On Becoming a Person*. Boston: Houghton Mifflin Co.

Rogers, C.R. (1969). *Freedom to Learn: A View of What Education Might Become*. Columbus, OH: Charles Merrill.

Rogers, M.E. (1980). Nursing: A Science of Unitary Man. In J.P. Riehl & C. Roy (Eds), *Conceptual Models for Nursing Practice*, 2nd Edn. (pp. 329–337). New York: AppletonCenturyCrofts.

Rosenthal, K.A. (1992). Coronary care patients' and nurses' perceptions of important nurse caring behaviors. *Heart & Lung*, 21, 536–539.

Royal College of Nursing (2003). *Defining Nursing*. London: Royal College of Nursing.

Royal College of Nursing (2004). *Nursing Assessment and Older People: A Royal College of Nursing Toolkit*. London: Royal College of Nursing.

Royal College of Nursing (1996). *Nursing Homes: Nursing Values*. London: Royal College of Nursing.

Royal College of Nursing (2007). *Workplace Resources for Practice Development*. London: Royal College of Nursing Institute.

Royal College of Nursing (2008). *Defending Dignity: Challenges and Opportunities for Nursing*. London: Royal College of Nursing.

Rycroft-Malone, J., Kitson, A., Harvey, G., McCormack, B., Seers, K., Titchen, A. & Estabrooks, C. (2002). Ingredients for change: revisiting a conceptual framework. *Quality and Safety in Health Care*, 11, 174–180. www.qualityhealthcare.com

Rycroft-Malone, J., Seers, K., Titchen, A., Harvey, G., Kitson, A. & McCormack, B. (2003). What counts as evidence in evidence-based practice. *Journal of Advanced Nursing*, 47(1), 81–90.

Rycroft-Malone, J., Harvey, G., Seers, K., Kitson, A.L., McCormack, B. & Titchen, A. (2004). An exploration of the factors that influence the implementation of evidence into practice. *Journal of Clinical Nursing*, 13(8), 913–924.

Sartre, J.P. (1972). *Being and Nothingness*. London: Methuen & Co. Ltd.

Schein, E.H. (2004). *Organizational Culture and Leadership*, 3rd Edn. San Franscisco: John Wiley & Sons Inc.

Schoenhofer, S.O. (2002). Choosing personhood: intentionality and the theory of nursing as caring. *Holistic Nursing Practice*, 16,(4), 36–40.

Schofield, I. (1994). An historical approach to care. *Elderly Care*, 6(6), 14–15.

Schon, D.A. (1983). *The Reflective Practitioner: How Professional Think in Action*. New York: Basic books.

Selder, F. (1989). Life transition theory: the resolution of uncertainty. *Nursing and Health Care*, 10(8), 437–451.

Senge, P. (2006). *The Fifth Discipline*. London: Random House Business Books.

Shaw, T. (2005). Leadership for Practice Development. In M. Jasper & M. Jumaa (Eds), *Effective Healthcare Leadership* (pp. 207–221). Oxford, UK: Blackwell Publishing Ltd.

Shaw, T., Dewing, J., Young, R., Devlin, M., Boomer, C. & Legius, M. (2008). Enabling Practice Development: Delving into the Concept of Facilitation from a Practitioner Perspective. In K. Manley, B. McCormack & V. Wilson (Eds), *International Practice Development in Nursing and Healthcare* (pp. 147–169). Oxford: Blackwell Publishing.

Slater, L. (2006). Person-centredness: a concept analysis. *Contemporary Nurse*, 23, 135–144.

Slater, P. (2006). Person Centred Nursing: The Development and Testing of a Valid and Reliable Nursing Outcomes Instrument. Unpublished PhD. University of Ulster, Jordanstown, Northern Ireland.

Slater, P., McCormack, B. & Bunting, B. (2009). The development and pilot testing of an instrument to measure nurses' working environment: the Nursing Context Index, *Worldviews on Evidence Based Nursing*, 6(3), 173–182.

Slater, P., O'Halloran, P., Connolly, D. & McCormack, B. (2009). Testing the factor structure of the Nursing Work Index – Revised, *Worldviews on Evidence Based Nursing*, 6(3): early view http://www3.interscience.wiley.com/journal/122523249/abstract.

Sloane, P.D., Hoeffer, B., Mitchell, C.M., McKenzie, D.A., Barrick, A.L., Rader, J., Stewart, B.J., Talerico, K.A., Rasin, J.H., Zink, R.C. & Koch, G.G. (2004). Effect of person-centred showering and the towel bath on bathing-associated aggression, agitation, and discomfort in nursing home residents with dementia: a randomized controlled trial. *Journal of the American Geriatric Society*, 52(11), 1797–1804.

Smith, F.B. (1982). *Florence Nightingale – Reputation and Power.* London: Taylor and Francis.

Spillsbury, K. & Meyer, J. (2001). Defining the nursing contribution to patient outcome: lessons learned from a review of the literature examining nursing outcomes, skill-mix and changing roles. *Journal of Clinical Nursing*, 10(1), 3–14.

Stamp, P.L. & Piedmonte, E.B. (1986). *Nurses and Work Satisfaction an Index of Measurement.* Lexington, MA: DC Heath.

Staniszewska, S. & Ahmed, L. (1999). The concepts of expectation and satisfaction: do they capture the way patients evaluate their care? *Journal of Advanced Nursing*, 29(2), 364–372.

Stevens-Barnum, B.J.S. (1994). *Nursing Theory: Analysis, Application, Evaluation*, 4th Edn. Philadelphia: J.B. Lippincott Company.

Stoddart, E. (1998). Dementia care: supporting a plea for personhood. *Scottish Journal of Healthcare Chaplaincy*, 1, 9–11.

Sullivan, R.J. (1990). *Immanuel Kant's Moral Theory.* Cambridge: Cambridge University Press.

Swanson, K.M. (1991). Empirical development of a middle range theory of caring. *Nursing Research*, 40(3), 161–166.

Swanson, K.M. (1993). Nursing as informed caring for the well-being of others. *Journal of Nursing Scholarship*, 25(4), 352–357.

Sykes, J.B. (1976). *The Concise Oxford Dictionary of Current English*, 6th Edn. Oxford: Clarendon Press.

Thomas, C., Ward, M., Chobra, C. & Kumiega, A. (1990). Measuring and interpreting organizational culture. *Journal of Nursing Administration*, 20(6), 17–24.

Titchen, A. (2001). Critical Companionship: A Conceptual Framework for Developing Expertise. In A. Higgs & A. Titchen (Eds), *Practice Knowledge and Expertise in the Health Professions*. Oxford: Butterworth Heinemann.

Titchen, A. (2004). Helping Relationships for Practice Development: Critical Companionship. In B. McCormack, K. Manley & R. Garbett (Eds), *Practice Development in Nursing*. Oxford: Blackwell.

Titchen, A. (2009). Developing Expertise through Nurturing Professional Artistry in the Workplace. In S. Hardy, A. Titchen, B. McCormack & K. Manley (Eds), *Revealing Nursing Expertise through Practitioner Inquiry*. Oxford: Wiley-Blackwell.

Titchen, A. & Binnie, A. (1995). The art of clinical supervision. *Journal of Clinical Nursing*, 4(5), 327–334.

Titchen, A. & McCormack, B. (2008). A Methodological Walk in the Forest: Critical Creativity and Human Flourishing. In K. Manley, B. McCormack & V. Wilson (Eds), *International Practice Development in Nursing and Healthcare* (pp. 59–83). Oxford: Blackwell.

Titchen, A. & McGinley, M. (2003). Facilitating practitioner research through critical companionship. *NTResearch*, 8(2), 115–131.

Tolson, D. (1999). Practice innovation: a methodological maze. *Journal of Advanced Nursing*, 30, 381–390.

Tonuma, M. & Wimbolt, M. (2000). From rituals to reason: creating an environment that allows nurses to nurse. *International Journal of Nursing Practice*, 6(4), 214–218.

Tournier, P. (1999). *Meaning of Persons.* London: SCM Press Ltd.

Tronto, J.C. (1993). *Moral Boundaries: A Political Argument for an Ethic of Care.* London: Routledge.

Turner-Stokes, L. (2007). Politics, policy and payment – facilitators or barriers to person-centred rehabilitation? *Disability and Rehabilitation*, 29(20–21), 1575–1582.

Tzeng, H.M., Ketefian, S. & Redman, R. (2002) Relationship of nurses' assessment of organisational culture, job satisfaction and patient satisfaction with nursing care. *International Journal of Nursing Studies* 39, 79–84.

United Kingdom Central Council for Nursing, Midwifery and Health Visiting (1992). *The Code of Professional Conduct.* London: UKCC.

Upenieks, V.V. (2002). Assessing differences in job satisfaction of nurses in magnet and non-magnet hospitals. *Journal of Nursing Administration,* 32(11), 564–576.

Vincent, J.L., Alexander, J.G., Money, B. & Patterson, M.S. (1996). How parents describe caring behaviors of nurses in pediatric intensive care. *American Journal of Maternal Children's Nursing,* 21, 197–201.

von Essen, L. & Sjoden, P.O. (1991). Patient and staff perceptions of caring: review and replication. *Journal of Advanced Nursing,* 16, 1363–1374.

Wagner, L. (1994). Innovation in Primary Health Care for Elderly People in Denmark: Two Action Research Projects. Thesis. The Nordic School of Public Health, Gothenbgurg, Sweden.

Walsh, M. & Dolan, B. (1999). Emergency nurses and their perceptions of caring. *Emergency Nurse,* 7(4), 24–31.

Walsh, K., Lawless, J., Moss, C. & Allbon, C. (2005). The development of an engagement tool for practice development. *Practice Development in Healthcare,* 4(3), 124–130.

Ward, P. (1997). *360 Degree Feedback.* London: Institute of Personnel and Development.

Warfield, C. & Manley, K. (1990). Developing a new philosophy in the NDU. *Nursing Standard,* 4(41), 27–30.

Warnock, M. (1970). *Existentialism.* London: Oxford University Press.

Watson, J. (1979). *Nursing: The Philosophy and Science of Caring.* Boston: Little Brown.

Watson, J. (1985). *Nursing: Human Science and Human Care – A Theory of Nursing.* New York: National League of Nursing Press.

Watson, R., Deary, I.J. & Lea, A. (1999). A longitudinal study into the perceptions of caring among student nurses using multivariate analysis of the caring dimensions inventory. *Journal of Advanced Nursing,* 30, 1080–1089.

Watson, R., Deary, I.J. & Hoogbruin, A.L. (2001). A 35-item version of the Caring Dimensions Index (CDI – 35): multivariate analysis and application to a longitudinal study involving student nurses. *International Journal of Nursing Studies,* 38, 511–521.

Watson, R., Deary, I.J., Lea Hoogbruin, A., Vermeijden, W., Rumeu, C., Beunza, M., Barbarin, B., MacDonald, J. & McCready, T. (2003a). Perceptions of nursing: a study involving nurses, nursing students, patients and non-nursing students. *International Journal of Nursing Studies,* 43, 133–144.

Watson, R., Lea Hoogbruin, A., Rumeu, C., Beunza, M., Barbarin, B., MacDonald, J. & McCready, T. (2003b). Differences and similarities in the perception of caring between Spanish and UK nurses. *Journal of Clinical Nursing,* 12, 85–92.

Webster, J. (2004). Person-centred assessment with older people. Person-centred assessment with older people. *Nursing Older People,* 16(3), 22–26.

Weisinger, H. (1998). *Emotional Intelligence at Work.* San Francisco: Jossey-Bass.

Wilkinson, J.R. (1998). What it means to care. *Curationis,* 21(2), 2–8.

Williams, C.L. & Tappen, R.M. (1999). Can we create a therapeutic relationship with nursing home residents in the later stages of Alzheimer's disease? *Journal of Psychosocial Nursing,* 37(3), 28–35.

Wilson, V. (2005). Developing a vision for teamwork. *Practice Development in Healthcare,* 4(1), 40–48.

Wilson, V., McCormack, B. & Ives, G. (2005). Understanding the workplace culture of a special care nursery. *Journal of Advanced Nursing*, 50(1), 27–38.

Wilson, V., McCormack, B. and Ives, G. (2006). Replacing the 'self' in learning. *Learning in Health and Social Care*, 5(2), 90–105.

Wilson, V., Hardy, S. & Brown, R. (2008). An Exploration of Practice Development Evaluation: Unearthing Praxis. In K. Manley, B. McCormack & V. Wilson (Eds), *Practice Development in Nursing: International Perspectives*. Oxford: Blackwell Publishing.

Woods, R.T. (2001). Discovering the person with Alzheimer's disease: cognitive, emotional and behavioural aspects. *Aging and Mental Health*, 5(supplement 1), S7–S16.

Woodward, V.M. (1997). Professional caring: a contradiction in terms? *Journal of Advanced Nursing*, 26, 999–1004.

Wright, J. & McCormack, B. (2001). Practice development: individualised care. *Nursing Standard*, 15(36), 37–42.

Wylie, K., Madjar, I. & Walton, J.A. (2002). Dementia care mapping: a person-centred, evidence-based approach to improving the quality of care in residential care settings. *Geriaction*, 20(2), 5–9.

Yegdich, T. (1999). On the phenomenology of empathy in nursing: empathy or sympathy? *Journal of Advanced Nursing*, 30(1), 83–93.

Younger, D. & Martin, G.W. (2000). Dementia care mapping: an approach to quality audit of services for people with dementia in two health districts. *Journal of Advanced Nursing*, 32(5), 1206–1212.

Index

Note: Page numbers in *italics* refer to figures and tables.

Keep up with critical fields

Would you like to receive up-to-date information on our books, journals and databases in the areas that interest you, direct to your mailbox?

Join the **Wiley e-mail service** - a convenient way to receive updates and exclusive discount offers on products from us.

Simply visit **www.wiley.com/email** and register online

We won't bombard you with emails and we'll only email you with information that's relevant to you. We will ALWAYS respect your e-mail privacy and NEVER sell, rent, or exchange your e-mail address to any outside company. Full details on our privacy policy can be found online.

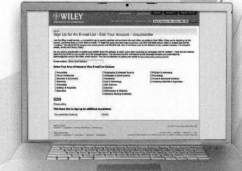

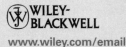

www.wiley.com/email